Multiple Sclerosis Rehabilitation

Editors

SHANA L. JOHNSON
GEORGE H. KRAFT

PHYSICAL MEDICINE AND REHABILITATION CLINICS OF NORTH AMERICA

www.pmr.theclinics.com

Consulting Editor
GREGORY T. CARTER

November 2013 • Volume 24 • Number 4

ELSEVIER

1600 John F. Kennedy Boulevard • Suite 1800 • Philadelphia, Pennsylvania, 19103-2899

http://www.theclinics.com

PHYSICAL MEDICINE AND REHABILITATION CLINICS OF NORTH AMERICA Volume 24, Number 4
November 2013 ISSN 1047-9651, ISBN 978-0-323-24233-2

Editor: Jessica McCool

Reprints. For copies of 100 or more of articles in this publication, please contact the Commercial Reprints Department, Elsevier Inc., 360 Park Avenue South, New York, NY 10010-1710. Tel.: 212-633-3874; Fax: 212-633-3820; E-mail: reprints@elsevier.com.

Physical Medicine and Rehabilitation Clinics of North America (ISSN 1047-9651) is published quarterly by Elsevier Inc., 360 Park Avenue South, New York, NY 10010-1710. Months of issue are February, May, August, and November. Business and Editorial Offices: 1600 John F. Kennedy Blvd., Suite 1800, Philadelphia, PA 19103-2899. Customer Service Office: 3251 Riverport Lane, Maryland Heights, MO 63043. Periodicals postage paid at New York, NY and additional mailing offices. Subscription price per year is $275.00 (US individuals), $486.00 (US institutions), $145.00 (US students), $335.00 (Canadian individuals), $640.00 (Canadian institutions), $210.00 (Canadian students), $415.00 (foreign individuals), $640.00 (foreign institutions), and $210.00 (foreign students). Foreign air speed delivery is included in all Clinics subscription prices. All prices are subject to change without notice. **POSTMASTER:** Send address changes to Physical Medicine and Rehabilitation Clinics of North America, Customer Service Office: Elsevier Health Sciences Division, Subscription Customer Service, 3251 Riverport Lane, Maryland Heights, MO 63043. **Customer Service: 1-800-654-2452 (US). From outside of the United States, call 314-447-8871. Fax: 314-447-8029. E-mail: JournalsCustomer Service-usa@elsevier.com (for print support); JournalsOnlineSupport-usa@elsevier.com (for online support).**

Physical Medicine and Rehabilitation Clinics of North America is indexed in Excerpta Medica, MEDLINE/ PubMed (Index Medicus), Cinahl, and Cumulative Index to Nursing and Allied Health Literature.

Printed and bound by CPI Group (UK) Ltd, Croydon, CR0 4YY

Transferred to digital print 2012

Contributors

CONSULTING EDITOR

GREGORY T. CARTER, MD, MS
Medical Director, St Luke's Rehabilitation Institute, Spokane, Washington

EDITORS

SHANA L. JOHNSON, MD
Assistant Professor, Department of Rehabilitation Medicine, University of Washington, Seattle, Washington

GEORGE H. KRAFT, MD, MS
Alvord Professor of MS Research, Department of Rehabilitation Medicine, University of Washington School of Medicine, University of Washington, Seattle, Washington

AUTHORS

KEVIN N. ALSCHULER, PhD
Acting Assistant Professor, Department of Rehabilitation Medicine, University of Washington School of Medicine, Seattle, Washington

DAGMAR AMTMANN, PhD
Professor, Department of Rehabilitation Medicine, University of Washington School of Medicine, Seattle, Washington

ALYSSA M. BAMER, MPH
Research Scientist, Department of Rehabilitation Medicine, University of Washington School of Medicine, Seattle, Washington

CHARLES H. BOMBARDIER, PhD
Professor, Department of Rehabilitation Medicine, University of Washington School of Medicine, Seattle, Washington

JULIE BRUNINGS, MS-CCC, BC-ANCDS
Speech and Language Pathologist, Rehabilitation Therapy Department, University of Washington Medical Center, Seattle, Washington

ANN BUZAID, MA, OTR/L, ATP
Manager, Department of Occupational Therapy, University of Washington Medical Center, Seattle, Washington

KARON F. COOK, PhD
Research Associate Professor, Department of Psychology, Northwestern University Feinberg School of Medicine, Chicago, Illinois

MARIE Y. DAVIS, MD, PhD
Senior Fellow, Department of Neurology, University of Washington, Seattle, Washington

MARY PAT DODGE, MS, OTR/L
Occupational Therapist II, Department of Occupational Therapy, University of Washington Medical Center, Seattle, Washington

DAWN M. EHDE, PhD
Professor, Department of Rehabilitation Medicine, University of Washington School of Medicine, Seattle, Washington

COURTNEY E. FRANCIS, MD
Assistant Professor, Neuro-Ophthalmology, Department of Ophthalmology, University of Washington, Seattle, Washington

ROBERT FRASER, PhD
Professor, Department of Rehabilitation Medicine, University of Washington School of Medicine, Seattle, Washington

MYRON GOLDBERG, PhD, ABPP-CN
Clinical Professor, Department of Rehabilitation Medicine, University of Washington School of Medicine, Seattle, Washington

KELLI GOODMAN, PT, DPT
University of Washington Medicine, Seattle, Washington

LYNNE HANDMACHER, OTR/L
Occupational Therapist, Private Contract Therapist, Private Practice, Tacoma, Washington

LYNDA HILLMAN, DNP, ARNP
Rehabilitation Medicine/Multiple Sclerosis Nurse Practitioner, Multiple Sclerosis Center, University of Washington Medical Center, Seattle, Washington

ILEANA M. HOWARD, MD
Clinical Assistant Professor, Department of Rehabilitation Medicine, University of Washington; Rehabilitation Care Services, Veteran Affairs Puget Sound Health Care System, Seattle, Washington

CHRISTINA HUGHES, MD
Department of Physical Medicine and Inpatient Neuro Rehabilitation, Virginia Mason Medical Center, Seattle, Washington

MARK P. JENSEN, PhD
Professor, Department of Rehabilitation Medicine, University of Washington School of Medicine, Seattle, Washington

KURT L. JOHNSON, PhD
Professor, Department of Rehabilitation Medicine, University of Washington School of Medicine, Seattle, Washington

PAMELA J. KILTZ, MOTR/L
Occupational Therapist II, Department of Occupational Therapy, University of Washington Medical Center, Seattle, Washington

JISEON KIM, PhD
Department of Rehabilitation Medicine, University of Washington, Seattle, Washington

GEORGE H. KRAFT, MD, MS
Alvord Professor of MS Research, Department of Rehabilitation Medicine, University of Washington School of Medicine, University of Washington, Seattle, Washington

PATRICIA K. OAKES, MD, JD
Assistant Professor, Department of Neurology, University of Washington, Seattle, Washington

MARY PEPPING, PhD, ABPP-CN
Professor, Department of Rehabilitation Medicine, University of Washington School of Medicine, Seattle, Washington

TONI S. RODDEY, PT, PhD, FAAOMPT
School of Physical Therapy, College of Health Sciences, Texas Woman's University, Houston, Texas

KATHERINE ROUGH, PT, DPT, NCS
University of Washington Medicine, Seattle, Washington

ALI SAMII, MD
Professor of Neurology, Department of Neurology, Seattle VA Medical Center, University of Washington, Seattle, Washington

ALEXIUS E.G. SANDOVAL, MD
Department of Rehabilitation Medicine, Eastern Maine Medical Center, Bangor, Maine

SINDHU R. SRIVATSAL, MD, MPH
Senior Fellow, Department of Neurology, University of Washington, Seattle, Washington

VICTORIA STEVENS, PT, NCS
University of Washington Medicine, Seattle, Washington

AIMEE M. VERRALL, MPH
Research Manager, Department of Rehabilitation Medicine, University of Washington School of Medicine, Seattle, Washington

CLAIRE C. YANG, MD
Professor of Urology, University of Washington, VA Puget Sound Health Care System, Seattle, Washington

KATHRYN YORKSTON, PhD
Professor, Department of Rehabilitation Medicine, University of Washington School of Medicine, Seattle, Washington

Contents

Foreword: Multiple Sclerosis Rehabilitation   xiii

Gregory T. Carter

Preface: Multiple Sclerosis Rehabilitation   xvii

Shana L. Johnson and George H. Kraft

Gait Impairment and Optimizing Mobility in Multiple Sclerosis   573

Victoria Stevens, Kelli Goodman, Katherine Rough, and George H. Kraft

Multiple sclerosis (MS) is an immune-mediated disease that causes demy-elination and degeneration within the brain and spinal cord. This may result in many impairments, including impaired ambulation, muscle weakness, abnormal tone, visual disturbances, decreased sensation, and fatigue. Rehabilitation helps patients with MS maximize independence by helping to manage and minimize impairments. Deficits seen in ambulation should be addressed to improve energy efficiency and reduce falls. Compensation through appropriate prescription of assistive devices, bracing, and wheelchairs will help improve safety. Rehabilitation can make a significant impact on achieving and maintaining quality of life and independence.

Spasticity Management in Multiple Sclerosis   593

Christina Hughes and Ileana M. Howard

Spasticity is a prevalent and potentially disabling symptom common in individuals with multiple sclerosis. Adequate evaluation and management of spasticity requires a careful assessment of the patient's history to deter-mine functional impact of spasticity and potential exacerbating factors, and physical examination to determine the extent of the condition and culpable muscles. A host of options for spasticity management are avail-able: therapeutic exercise, physical modalities, complementary/alternative medicine interventions, oral medications, chemodenervation, and implan-tation of an intrathecal baclofen pump. Choice of treatment hinges on a combination of the extent of symptoms, patient preference, and avail-ability of services.

Exercise in Multiple Sclerosis   605

Alexius E.G. Sandoval

Exercise is an intervention that may be used in the management of multiple sclerosis (MS). Certain exercise physiology characteristics are commonly seen among persons with MS, particularly in the more debilitated. Studies have shown that properly prescribed exercise programs can improve modifiable impairments in MS. Exercise is generally safe and well toler-ated. General guidelines are available for exercise prescription for the MS population. There are several recommendations that may help improve the quality of future MS exercise trials.

Caregiving in Multiple Sclerosis   619

Lynda Hillman

Thirty percent of persons with multiple sclerosis (pwMS) require caregiving owing to their disability, and 80% of care to pwMS is provided by informal unpaid caregivers. The average caregiver is male, in a spousal/partner relationship with the pwMS, and provides more than 4 hours per day of care for many years. The physical, emotional, and time-intensive nature of caregiving for pwMS frequently impairs the caregiver's own physical and emotional health. Rehabilitation medicine professionals should be aware of the high risk of caregiver burden. Assessment of caregiver needs and appropriate intervention will help minimize the burden on caregivers.

Activities of Daily Living: Evaluation and Treatment in Persons with Multiple Sclerosis   629

Ann Buzaid, Mary Pat Dodge, Lynne Handmacher, and Pamela J. Kiltz

Symptoms of multiple sclerosis can create mild to severe changes in a person's abilities to perform activities of daily living. Occupational therapy assessment and treatment of impairments related to movement, sensory-related symptoms, fatigue, and cognitive impairments can have a significant impact on the quality of life of persons with multiple sclerosis.

Movement Disorders in Multiple Sclerosis   639

Patricia K. Oakes, Sindhu R. Srivatsal, Marie Y. Davis, and Ali Samii

Movement disorders constitute a subspecialty of neurology focusing on a variety of conditions characterized by hypokinetic, hyperkinetic, or abnormally coordinated movements including, among others, tremor, dystonia, parkinsonism, myoclonus, chorea, ballismus, tics, restless limbs, and ataxia. The term "movement disorders" may be used to refer to either abnormal movements or syndromes that cause these abnormal movements. The classification of movement disorders is based on phenomenology, individual syndromes, or etiology. This article reviews terminology used to describe movement disorders, discusses individual movement disorders and their occurrence in patients with multiple sclerosis, and reviews treatment options.

Multiple Sclerosis and Fatigue: Understanding the Patient's Needs   653

Karon F. Cook, Alyssa M. Bamer, Toni S. Roddey, George H. Kraft, Jiseon Kim, and Dagmar Amtmann

Fatigue is among the most common and debilitating symptoms of multiple sclerosis (MS), affecting approximately 80% of persons who have the disease. Recently, as part of the National Institutes of Health Patient Reported Outcome Measurement Information System (PROMIS), a bank of items was developed for measuring self-reported fatigue. This article has two purposes. (1) To assess, from the perspective of individuals living with MS, the relevance of a subset of items from the PROMIS fatigue item bank. (2) To identify additional aspects of fatigue that individuals with MS believe are important for clinicians when asking about their fatigue experience.

Cognition, Cognitive Dysfunction, and Cognitive Rehabilitation in Multiple
Sclerosis   663

Mary Pepping, Julie Brunings, and Myron Goldberg

> This article focuses on approaches and techniques for effective cognitive
> rehabilitation with people who have multiple sclerosis (MS). The patterns
> of preserved versus disrupted neuropsychological functions are reviewed.
> The relevant brain anatomy and physiology that underlie the common neu-
> rocognitive and neurobehavioral changes are described. The essential
> role is highlighted of comprehensive neuropsychological, speech lan-
> guage pathology, and clinical evaluations in the design and refinements
> of cognitive retraining treatment. The functional impact of cognitive
> problems expected with MS is emphasized, accompanied by examples
> of cognitive retraining approaches used to manage them and improve
> day-to-day performance.

Bladder Management in Multiple Sclerosis   673

Claire C. Yang

> This article reviews the basic principles and therapeutic options in the
> management of the neurogenic bladder due to multiple sclerosis (MS),
> written primarily for the non-urology provider. An algorithm for the initial
> management of the MS patient with lower urinary tract symptoms is
> provided.

Visual Issues in Multiple Sclerosis   687

Courtney E. Francis

> Multiple sclerosis has several ophthalmic manifestations, including optic
> neuritis, internuclear ophthalmoplegia, and nystagmus. The presentation,
> treatment, and prognosis of visual complaints secondary to multiple scle-
> rosis are discussed. Additionally, the use of optical coherence tomography
> and complications related to the use of fingolimod are considered.

Co-occurring Depression and Pain in Multiple Sclerosis   703

Kevin N. Alschuler, Dawn M. Ehde, and Mark P. Jensen

> Depression and pain are highly prevalent among individuals with multiple
> sclerosis, and they often co-occur. The purpose of this article is to summa-
> rize the literature and theory related to the comorbidity of pain and depres-
> sion and describe how their presence can impact individuals with multiple
> sclerosis. Additionally, the article discusses how existing treatments of
> pain and depression could be adapted to address shared mechanisms
> and overcome barriers to treatment utilization.

Evoked Potentials in Multiple Sclerosis   717

George H. Kraft

> Before the development of magnetic resonance imaging (MRI), evoked
> potentials (EPs)—visual evoked potentials, somatosensory evoked poten-
> tials, and brain stem auditory evoked responses—were commonly used to
> determine a second site of disease in patients being evaluated for possible
> multiple sclerosis (MS). The identification of an area of the central nervous

system showing abnormal conduction was used to supplement the abnormal signs identified on the physical examination—thus identifying the "multiple" in MS. This article is a brief overview of additional ways in which central nervous system (CNS) physiology—as measured by EPs—can still contribute value in the management of MS in the era of MRIs.

Future Directions of Multiple Sclerosis Rehabilitation Research   721

George H. Kraft, Kurt L. Johnson, Dagmar Amtmann, Alyssa M. Bamer, Charles H. Bombardier, Dawn M. Ehde, Robert Fraser, Aimee M. Verrall, and Kathryn Yorkston

Multiple sclerosis continues to present a host of rehabilitation challenges, specifically the impact of secondary "hidden" conditions on quality of life, participation, and employment. To discuss the current state of rehabilitation research and direct future research endeavors, a state of the science conference was held in November 2010 in Alexandria, Virginia. The conference was presented by the University of Washington's Multiple Sclerosis Rehabilitation Research and Training Center and focused on the current state of research into secondary conditions, outcomes measurement, employment, and the utility of psychotherapeutic interventions. This article discusses the details and recommendations of this conference.

Index   731

PHYSICAL MEDICINE & REHABILITATION CLINICS OF NORTH AMERICA

FORTHCOMING ISSUES

February 2014
Amputee Rehabilitation
Robert H. Meier III, MD, *Editor*

May 2014
Challenging Pain Syndromes
Adam L. Schreiber, DO,
Editor

August 2014
Spinal Cord Injury Rehabilitation
Diana Cardenas, MD, MHA and
Kevin Dalal, MD, *Editors*

RECENT ISSUES

August 2013
Life Care Planning
Michel Lacerte, MDCM, MSc, FRCPC, CCRC
and Cloie B. Johnson, MEd, ABVE-D, CCM,
Editors

May 2013
**Ambulation in Adults with Central
Neurologic Disorders**
Francois Bethoux, MD, *Editor*

February 2013
**The Electrodiagnosis of Neuromuscular
Disorders**
Michael D. Weiss, MD, *Editor*

RELATED INTEREST

Neurologic Clinics, February 2013 (Vol. 31, Issue 1)
Spinal Cord Diseases
Alireza Minagar, MD, FAAN and Alejandro A. Rabinstein, MD, FAAN, *Editors*
http://www.neurologic.theclinics.com/

VISIT THE CLINICS ONLINE!
Access your subscription at:
www.theclinics.com

NOW AVAILABLE FOR YOUR iPhone and iPad

Foreword

Multiple Sclerosis Rehabilitation

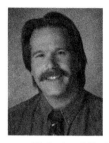

Gregory T. Carter, MD, MS
Consulting Editor

This issue is guest edited by Dr Shana Johnson along with her mentor, Dr George Kraft. Dr Johnson was hand-picked by Dr Kraft to be the new and current director of the University of Washington Medicine Multiple Sclerosis Center here in Seattle, Washington. Indeed, as his protégé and former fellow, she is well on her way to following in his footsteps. Thus, we have the best possible guest editors for this issue, and they have recruited a truly distinguished group of authors. Most of you know that Dr Kraft was the previous consulting medical editor for the *Physical Medicine and Rehabilitation Clinics of North America*, having held that position for over 30 years. Last year, Dr Kraft passed the honor of this editorship on to me and I am striving to keep up with his legacy of excellence in keeping the *Physical Medicine and Rehabilitation Clinics of North America* a Medline-referenced source of cutting-edge clinical reviews. Having Drs Johnson and Kraft as guest editors continues that tradition of excellence indeed.

In our field of physiatry, a sentence containing the words "multiple sclerosis" and "rehabilitation" will likely also include the name "Dr George Kraft." George has received just about every major award there is in the field of multiple sclerosis research, including the prestigious Lifetime Achievement Award from the National Multiple Sclerosis Society. I suspect there will be many future awards for Dr Johnson as she continues to build on the foundation built by Dr Kraft.

Here in the Pacific Northwest, multiple sclerosis (or MS) is fairly common, yet it is still shocking to me how disabling this disease may be as it attacks the central nervous system, whether relentlessly or sporadically. New pharmacological treatments have helped considerably, but still it is **rehabilitation modalities** that translate disease modification from a drug into actual improvement in **functionality**. This issue of the *Physical Medicine and Rehabilitation Clinics of North America* provides you with all the information a practicing physiatrist will need to provide the optimal care for a patient battling MS.

Phys Med Rehabil Clin N Am 24 (2013) xiii–xv
http://dx.doi.org/10.1016/j.pmr.2013.07.005
1047-9651/13/$ – see front matter © 2013 Published by Elsevier Inc.

The first article, "Gait Impairment and Optimizing Mobility in Multiple Sclerosis," is authored by Dr Kraft along with senior MS physical therapists, Victoria Stevens, Kelli Goodman, and Katherine Rough. In this article, you will find detailed information on how to maximize ambulatory skills in someone with MS.

Drs Christina Hughes and Ileana Howard provide us with an article entitled, "Spasticity Management in Multiple Sclerosis." Frankly, this is one of the best, most concise treatises on this topic I have ever read. This level of excellence is followed by another concise and very clinically useful discourse on "Exercise in Multiple Sclerosis," authored by Dr Alexius E.G. Sandoval, a noted MS expert and former MS fellow trained by Dr Kraft.

Lynda Hillman, DNP, does a wonderful job of reviewing all of the important aspects of "Caregiving in Multiple Sclerosis," going over perhaps one of the most important topics in terms of maintaining quality of life for these patients.

Again, a group of senior MS therapists, Ann Buzaid, Mary Pat Dodge, Lynne Handmacher, and Pamela J. Kiltz, gives us an excellent article on "Activities of Daily Living: Evaluation and Treatment in Persons with Multiple Sclerosis." This is remarkably thorough and has directly usable information.

My friend and noted expert on movement disorders, Dr Ali Samii, joins colleagues, Patricia K. Oakes, Sindhu R. Srivatsal, and Marie Y. Davis, to provide a thorough, up-to-date article on "Movement Disorders in Multiple Sclerosis." Following this, Dr Kraft and colleagues, Karon F. Cook, Alyssa M. Bamer, Toni S. Roddey, Jiseon Kim, and my friend, Dagmar Amtmann, review and update a hugely important topic, "Multiple Sclerosis and Fatigue: Understanding the Patient's Needs." Fatigue is one of the most common complaints in this patient population.

Mary Pepping, Julie Brunings, and Myron Goldberg give us an excellent update on "Cognition, Cognitive Dysfunction, and Cognitive Rehabilitation in Multiple Sclerosis." In this article, I most liked the specific management recommendations, as this is an area I always find particularly challenging.

Urologist Dr Claire C. Yang updates us on "Bladder Management in Multiple Sclerosis." Claire has tremendous expertise in managing complex rehabilitation patients with mixed functioning bladders.

Visual disturbances are often the presenting complaint in MS and Dr Courtney E. Francis provides us with a pertinent and directly useful piece on "Visual Issues in Multiple Sclerosis."

My close friend and research partner, Dr Mark Jensen, along with colleagues, Kevin N. Alschuler and Dawn M. Ehde, provide an outstanding discourse on "Co-Occurring Depression and Pain in Multiple Sclerosis." Dr Jensen and his group at the University of Washington are doing the absolute best work in this area and the value of their contributions to studying pain in the chronically disabled patient populations cannot be overstated.

No one understands "Evoked Potentials in Multiple Sclerosis" better than our editor here, Dr George H. Kraft. There is simply no one else who could have written this better—enough said.

Finally, we have a fantastic closing article, "Future Directions of Multiple Sclerosis Rehabilitation Research," written by a much-esteemed group, including many friends and colleagues. The group is led by Dr Kraft, along with Kurt L. Johnson, PhD, Dagmar Amtmann, PhD, Alyssa Bamer, MPH, Charles H. Bombardier, PhD, Dawn Ehde, PhD, Robert Fraser, PhD, Aimee M. Verrall, MPH, and Kathryn Yorkston, PhD. That is a powerful group of authors!

I would like to personally thank all of the authors who contributed to this issue and the countless hours they spent preparing these articles. Thanks to their efforts and perseverance, we are provided with a fantastic addition to the *Physical Medicine and Rehabilitation Clinics of North America*. Reading this issue is truly like reading the script for a prestigious MS fellowship!

Gregory T. Carter, MD, MS
St. Luke's Rehabilitation Institute
711 South Cowley Street
Spokane, WA 99202, USA

E-mail address:
gtcarter@uw.edu

Preface

Multiple Sclerosis Rehabilitation

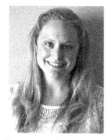 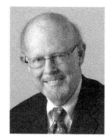

Shana L. Johnson, MD   George H. Kraft, MD, MS
Editors

This is the fourth issue of the *Physical Medicine and Rehabilitation Clinics of North America* on multiple sclerosis (MS) and it is the first one published under the direction of the new consulting editor, Gregory T. Carter, MD. As many of the long-time readers of the *Physical Medicine and Rehabilitation Clinics of North America* may recall, since I started this series in the early 1990s, and for its first 30+ years, I tried to publish issues on popular topics fairly often, and repeat other, but important topics, at least every seven years or so. At four issues of *Physical Medicine and Rehabilitation Clinics of North America* publishing per year, this resulted in revisiting a disease topic every 25 to 30 issues.

So it is time again for an issue on MS. I thank Dr Carter for asking Dr Shana Johnson and me to guest edit this issue and find myself in the unusual position of writing a Preface—not a Foreword—as I had done for over 30 years. Shana Johnson, MD, is the Co-Director of the University of Washington MS Center, and an Assistant Professor in the Department of Rehabilitation Medicine at the university. Dr Johnson had her PM&R residency at UT Southwestern in Dallas, and her MS Fellowship training program at the University of Washington. After a period of practice in Olympia, Washington—the state capital—where she established an MS clinic, we were fortunate to recruit her back to the UW to become Co-director of the UW MS Clinic.

How does this issue differ from the previous three issues on MS? One answer is obvious: understanding and management of MS are rapidly evolving—arguably faster than any other disorder followed by physiatrists. The understanding of the mechanism of MS, awareness that the disease actually represents more than one disease having different etiologies and mechanisms, new DMTs, the advent of the first "physiatric drug" (dalfampridine—Ampyra), which can improve walking in patients with MS, are all advances not known at the time of the publication of the last MS issue.

Phys Med Rehabil Clin N Am 24 (2013) xvii–xviii
http://dx.doi.org/10.1016/j.pmr.2013.07.004
1047-9651/13/$ – see front matter © 2013 Published by Elsevier Inc.

pmr.theclinics.com

Many of these advances are covered in this issue. But perhaps the greatest deviation from previous MS issues is noted in the title: "Rehabilitation." This issue is the first MS issue dedicated solely to the rehabilitation of MS. I thank Dr Shana Johnson for her shepherding of this issue to make it the definitive text on MS rehabilitation. And again, I want to thank Dr Greg Carter for asking us to be co-guest editors.

Shana L. Johnson, MD
Department of Rehabilitation Medicine
University of Washington
1959 NE Pacific Street
Seattle, WA 98195-6490, USA

George H. Kraft, MD, MS
Rehabilitation Medicine
University of Washington
Box 356490, 1959 Northeast Pacific Street
Seattle, WA 98195-6490, USA

E-mail addresses:
sljohnso@uw.edu (S.L. Johnson)
ghkraft@uw.edu (G.H. Kraft)

Gait Impairment and Optimizing Mobility in Multiple Sclerosis

Victoria Stevens, PT, NCS*, Kelli Goodman, PT, DPT,
Katherine Rough, PT, DPT, NCS, George H. Kraft, MD, MS

KEYWORDS

• Multiple sclerosis • Gait • Falls • Balance • Rehabilitation

KEY POINTS

- Multiple sclerosis (MS) is an immune-mediated disease that causes demyelination and axonal degeneration within the brain and spinal cord.
- Impairments include impaired ambulation, muscle weakness, abnormal tone, visual disturbances, decreased sensation, and fatigue.
- Rehabilitation helps patients with MS maximize independence by helping to manage and minimize impairments.
- Deficits seen in ambulation should be addressed to improve energy efficiency and reduce falls.
- Compensation through appropriate prescription of assistive devices, bracing, and wheelchairs will help improve safety.
- Rehabilitation can make a significant impact on achieving and maintaining quality of life and independence.

INTRODUCTION

Multiple sclerosis (MS) is an immune-mediated disease that causes both demyelination and axonal degeneration within the brain and spinal cord. These pathologic changes in the nerves of the central nervous system (CNS) may cause many impairments, commonly including muscle weakness, increased tone, bladder dysfunction, cognitive impairment, visual impairment, sensory changes, and fatigue. One of the signature characteristics of MS is its predilection for affecting muscles and sensation innervated by the most caudal nerves: muscles and sensory structures of the feet, legs, and bladder. This is because of the cumulative impact of lesions throughout the CNS; nerve dysfunction is greatest over the longest pathways: those between the cortex and lower lumbo-sacral roots (the "cumulative impact" explanation).[1]

There are currently a number of medications approved by the Food and Drug Administration (FDA) that can reduce the number of exacerbations and slow disease

University of Washington Medicine, Seattle, WA, USA
* Corresponding author.
E-mail address: vstevens@u.washington.edu

Phys Med Rehabil Clin N Am 24 (2013) 573–592
http://dx.doi.org/10.1016/j.pmr.2013.07.002
1047-9651/13/$ – see front matter © 2013 Elsevier Inc. All rights reserved.

progression (disease-modifying treatments or DMTs) and one medication that may improve walking (dalfampridine [Ampyra]), none of them provide a cure.[2] Rehabilitation aimed at maximizing patients' current levels of function and increasing their overall independence is an important adjunct to DMTs in MS care.[3]

GAIT ABNORMALITIES

Patients with MS have a range of gait abnormalities, including decreased step length, decreased cadence, reduced joint movement, and increased variability of most gait parameters. These changes lead to decreased velocity, reduced endurance, increased metabolic costs, and reduced community ambulation.[4] Even in those individuals with minimal disability (expanded disability status scale [EDSS] $\leq$3.5),[5] analysis shows that persons with MS walk slower, with fewer, shorter, wider steps; have increased variability in time between steps; and spend more time in double support compared with controls.[6]

Several types of abnormal gait patterns can arise as a result of MS; the specific pattern is dependent on the location of the lesions within the CNS. Some of the more common gait patterns are described in the following section and include spastic paresis, cerebellar ataxia, and sensory ataxia. Often a combination of patterns is seen.

Gait Patterns

Spastic paresis
Spastic paresis results from insufficient supraspinal recruitment of motor neurons in specific leg muscles during the gait cycle. Depending on which muscles are weak, limitations can be seen in stance or swing phase resulting in a variety of impairments including foot drop (ankle-foot weakness); knee hyperextension or hyperflexion; anterior, posterior, or lateral trunk lean; circumduction; and hip drop.[7] The most common pattern in MS is asymmetric spastic paraparesis, but all patterns can be seen, including monoparesis, hemiparesis, and tetraparesis.

Ankle-foot weakness in its mildest and most common form, it is manifested by 2 characteristics:

1. Weakness of ankle dorsiflexion (and sometimes associated weak push-off)
2. Motor fatigue

Motor fatigue is greater weakness with greater duration of use and is also accounted for by the likelihood of increased sequential demyelinated regions encountered over the longest pathways in the CNS. This is caused by conduction block seen in partially demyelinated motor pathways over an extended period of activation, and may be associated with increase in body temperature or other causes.[8] An easy assessment of this condition is to observe the wear pattern on the front of the sole of a shoe.

Cerebellar ataxia
Cerebellar ataxia occurs as a result of damage to the cerebellum or its connections and is characterized by incoordination, poor postural control, dysmetria, dysdiadochokinesia, and increased variability in stride length, as well as wide base of support and stooped trunk position.[6]

Sensory ataxia
Sensory ataxia results from damage to the dorsal columns of the spinal cord that transmit proprioception, or from damage in the processing centers for afferent information, such as the thalamus or the parietal lobe. This gait is characterized by postural instability, heavy heel strikes, poor kinematics from lower limb joint position, and

decreased gait velocity. This may be tested in clinic with the Romberg test: the patients with MS is asked to stand, feet together, and can do so with eyes open but not when closed. A more quantitative method of assessing posterior column function is with tibial nerve somatosensory evoked potentials (SEPs) (see the article by Kraft elsewhere in this issue for further exploration of this topic).[9]

Weakness

Overall muscle force generated during a contraction is lower in patients with MS because of reduced central motor drive and consequent muscle recruitment, reduced muscle metabolic response, and muscle atrophy due to disuse. Strength training is known to promote neural adaptations, such as improved motor unit activation and synchronization of firing rates, both of which deteriorate rapidly with inactivity.[7]

Strength training has been shown to be beneficial in several MS studies. Guitierrez and colleagues[10] showed that an 8-week program of resistance training improved gait kinematics. The study found that resistance training facilitates positive changes in gait (specifically, longer strides), more time spent in swing phase, and less time in the stance and double-support phase. This study also showed improved toe clearance, which is a significant factor in decreasing falls. A trend toward improvement in the self-reported EDSS scale, which relies heavily on ambulation as a determinant of disability, was also documented.[10] Kraft and colleagues[11] found improved function, strength, and psychosocial well-being in a group of patients with MS after a 3-month course of strength training. DeBolt and McCubbin[12] found that a home-based resistance program was well tolerated, caused no exacerbations in this population, and improved leg extension muscle power. This research demonstrates the critical importance of initiating an individualized home exercise program in a patient with MS. It is important that these patients are referred to physical therapy early on in their disease process to maximize strength and independence. Rehabilitation can make a significant impact on achieving and maintaining quality of life and independence.

Spasticity

Spasticity is commonly seen in the MS population. An increased level of tone is associated with higher levels of disability. Barnes and colleagues[13] investigated the prevalence of spasticity in 68 subjects and identified that 97% had spasticity in at least one leg that was present at a clinically significant level in 47%.

There are several muscles that commonly interfere with ambulation in the MS population. Hypertonic plantarflexors cause the foot to point down, making toe clearance in the swing phase of gait difficult, resulting in "catching the toe" and falling. Increased spasticity in the quadriceps muscles makes bending the knee during the swing phase and advancing the leg difficult. Hip adductors are also commonly affected, creating a scissoring gait. Increased tone in the hamstrings makes it difficult for the knee to be fully extended at midstance, limiting leg swing advancement, and causing the patient to bear weight on a bent knee. This increases the risk for knee buckling and results in decreased weight bearing, shorter step length, and decreased stance time on the affected limb.[7,14]

Fatigue

We were the first to describe fatigue as a symptom of MS,[15,16] and have identified it as the patents' most common symptom, occurring in 77% of patients with MS. Exercises and ambulation should be spread throughout the day, and the time of day can be an important factor in the success of the patient's exercise program. Patients with MS also report greater fatigue in warmer climates, because of heat sensitivity.[16] Cooling jackets, increased hydration, fans, air conditioners, and showers are all important strategies to maintaining a cooler core temperature to help reduce this.

Balance

Many people with MS have poor balance, resulting in frequent falls. Balance requires the integration of 3 sensory systems, visual, somatosensory, and vestibular, which inform the body about where it is in space, as well as its direction of movement and relationship to the environment.[17,18]

Visual system

The visual system provides information about how the body moves in its environment as well as allowing it to avoid obstacles.[17,19] With proprioceptive deficits, vision can be used as a substitution to preserve balance.

Somatosensory system

This system provides the brain information regarding location of the body and limbs in space, pressure and force exertion, and direction of limb movement.[17-19] Because of the "cumulative impact" (see earlier in this article) proprioception from the lower limbs is the most frequently involved afferent system in MS, and is the most common cause of imbalance in MS.[17]

Vestibular system

The vestibular system coordinates eye and head movements and assists with balance.[17] It is involved with ocular reflexes and a complex canal system that informs the brain about head position relative to gravity and angular/linear velocity.[14,17,19-21] Vestibular disorders are associated with vertigo (an illusion of movement, a spinning sensation), imbalance, inability to maintain stable gaze during head movement, and gait ataxia.[14,17,19]

Balance deficits

Balance during stance and gait requires central sensory integration of 3 sensory systems with suitable motor activity and sensorimotor changes that fluctuate based on body position, intention, and the environment. Central integration of sensory information in the cortex results in a coordinated motor output of the head, arms, legs, and trunk, and is used to control the center of mass in reaction to perturbations that are either self-generated in anticipation of movement or are caused externally.[14,17-19] If there is interruption in this communication, balance deficits are often seen. In a 2010 literature review by Cameron and Lord,[22] the mechanisms underlying imbalance in MS, such as changes in postural control, are likely primarily the result of slowed somatosensory conduction and impaired central integration, as opposed to being a result of cerebellar lesions.

Patients with MS demonstrate a decreased ability to stand still when compared with healthy controls, as evidenced by increased postural sway when their eyes are closed or base of support is decreased.[22] Huisingaa and colleagues also found that patients with MS have increased sway in both the anterior/posterior and mediolateral directions. In MS, it is possible that poor integration of vestibular information and slowed somatosensory feedback lead to the increased sway variability.

Patients with MS demonstrate slowed and shortened movement when reaching or stepping forward toward their limits of stability, and they have decreased ability to control anterior/posterior sway in response to unanticipated balance disturbances and perturbations.[22,23] Krishnan and colleagues[23] uncovered the underlying impairments in anticipatory postural control showing that compared with healthy controls, patients with MS have decreased and delayed anticipatory postural adjustments (APAs), as well as an increased backward compensation of center of pressure (CoP) displacement when reaching. These delays in APAs could be attributed to poor information processing in the CNS, but research has also shown they could be the result of delayed somatosensory conduction in the spine.[22,23]

Balance intervention

Studies have evaluated the efficacy of a variety of interventions for improving balance in patients with MS. Based on Cameron and Lord's[22] literature review, interventions related to sensory facilitation and dual-task practice are most effective. These specifically address the proprioceptive and central integration deficits that trigger imbalance and falls in patients with MS.[22] Task-specific, dual-task training has been used in various neurologic patient populations to improve postural control and has been hypothesized to be effective in patients with MS.[24] It is most effective when done in massed, variable, and random practice to promote neuroplasticity.[7] Therapy that focuses on sensory facilitation and integration provides controlled sensory input from the vestibular, tactile, and proprioceptive systems.[7] The retraining of sensory strategies may be an important way to recover both static and dynamic balance. Interventions specifically intended to improve balance or balance-related tasks show better results when compared with lower extremity strengthening or aerobic exercises.[25]

There is also research to support vestibular rehabilitation of patients with MS, with or without vestibular symptoms. Both Zeigelboim and colleagues[26] and Pavan and colleagues[20] showed that the use of vestibular exercises in treatment of patients with dizziness and relapsing-remitting MS was able to produce a small, significant change in balance and decreased disability via the Dizziness Handicap Inventory. Herbert and colleagues[27] demonstrated in a single-blinded, randomized controlled trial that vestibular rehabilitation exercises were an effective tool to decrease fatigue, improve postural control, and reduce disability in patients with MS with or without dizziness. Patients performed a 6-week progressive vestibular rehabilitation program focused on standing and half-kneeling balance activities that also incorporated eye, head, and body movements.[27] Herbert and colleagues[27] hypothesized that because postural control and dizziness reflect central processing, further support is lent to the idea that impairments of central sensory processing also contribute to fatigue in patients with MS.

Recent preliminary research provides insight into potentially beneficial intervention strategies for balance training in patients with MS. An 8-week core exercise program was shown to improve balance and gait in 62% of a small sample of patients with MS.[28] Preliminary research on the effect of therapeutic horseback riding and hippotherapy in patients with MS has shown potential for improved postural stability and gait, although further research is required.[29,30] There is also promising research on the incorporation of the Nintendo Wii Fit in the prescription of balance exercise programs.[31] Balance-based torso weighting, which involves small, subtle weighting of the trunk for improved upright mobility and to decrease ataxia, has also been researched. Studies have shown that this can be effective and demonstrates immediate improvements in gait velocity and functional activity.[32,33] Overall, further study and research is needed to fully determine the best recommendations for effective balance interventions in patients with MS.

Falls

Falls are common in persons with MS, with 1-time fall prevalence reported retrospectively between 50.5% and 58.2% and prospectively between 52.0% to 63.0% in studies collecting information on fall prevalence greater than 2 months.[34–44] Patients who have had 2+ falls demonstrate a prevalence retrospectively between 27.9% and 64.0%, and prospectively between 35.0% and 43.0%, indicating that the incidence of multiple falls in the MS population is extremely common.[35,37–43]

Peterson and colleagues[35] reported 50% of falls were injurious with 23% requiring medical care. Similar results were found by Matsuda and colleagues[42] with 58.5% and 18.9% respectively. Another study by Matsuda and colleagues[41] reported that 18.5% of fallers sought medical attention, whereas a study by Nilsagard and colleagues[37] found a higher number of 26.6%.[37,41] Cameron and colleagues[45] found a smaller number of veterans with MS had injurious falls at 2.8%. Interestingly, Kasser and colleagues[38] demonstrated that 81% of 1-time fallers reported injury, whereas recurrent fallers reported less injury at 47%. Differences in self-report were found in 1-time fallers, with falls more related to extrinsic environmental factors rather than the intrinsic disease-process–oriented falls found in recurrent fallers.

The study by Kasser and colleagues[38] is not the only one to examine differences between 1-time fallers and recurrent fallers. Matsuda and colleagues[42] also found significant differences in factors related to falling, suggesting that 1-time fallers are a distinct group from both nonfallers and recurrent fallers. However, across all groups, only 50.9% of people who fell reported discussing falls with a health care provider (HCP), and having an injurious fall or one requiring medical attention did not increase the likelihood of reporting these falls. Ninety-four percent of these reported falls were met with generalized fall-prevention strategy advice, suggesting that a more focused fall history discussion or individualized prevention strategies may increase the efficacy of fall reduction. For HCP to understand how to reduce falls, it is important to understand the multiple factors showed to be related to falls in MS (**Table 1**).

In addition to the findings in **Table 1**, falls in patients with MS have been found to be associated with low economic status,[42] infratentorial lesions,[39] environmental factors,[46] impaired central integration of afferent information,[22] temperature,[46] osteoporosis,[35] and poor mental health.[36,43] The relationship between falls and other factors, such as transfer ability,[42,46,47] fall history,[35,36,42,47] use of a wheelchair,[34–36,42] ability in activities of daily living,[36,47] and the role of vision[34,40,42,46] has demonstrated variable results in previous studies. Accumulation of body impairments[41] and medications[37] have been studied but thus far have not been shown to be associated with increased risk for falls.

Fear of falling (FoF) is common in patients with MS, with studies indicating a range of 41.1% to 60.0% of fallers reporting FoF.[34,37,41] However, FoF is not limited to fallers, as FoF is also reported in 25.9% to 68.0% of nonfallers.[37,41] FoF can also lead to activity curtailment, as was shown in a study by Peterson and colleagues,[36] in which 63.5% of both groups reported FoF and 82.6% of fallers and 46.6% of nonfallers limited their activity as a result. Activity curtailment related to FoF has been demonstrated in other studies with 42.9% to 8.8% and 27.7% to 71.4% of fallers and nonfallers reporting limiting their activity due to FoF respectively.

Few studies have looked at fall prevention and treatment of falls in MS. Finlayson and colleagues[50] suggested a 12-hour discussion group entitled "Safe at Home BAASE," focusing on increasing knowledge and skills for fall risk management and behavior modification to reduce fall risk. Results demonstrated participants reported gains in knowledge, skills, and behaviors to improve management of risk factors for falls.[50] Cattaneo and colleagues[26] studied groups of patients with MS receiving 12 sessions of motor balance training with and without emphasis on sensory balance training versus conservative therapy. Results showed both balance training groups significantly improved dynamic and static balance reducing falls. Coote and colleagues[43] found a 10-week group class focused on balance and strength significantly

Table 1
Reasons for falls in multiple sclerosis

Reason for Falls	Nilsagard et al,[37] 2009	Finlayson et al,[34] 2006	Matsuda et al,[42] 2011	Peterson et al,[35] 2008	Sosnoff et al,[40] 2011	Coote et al,[43] 2012	Nilsagard et al,[46] 2009	Kasser et al,[38] 2011	Cattaneo et al,[47,48] 2002	Prosperini et al,[39] 2011	Peterson et al,[36] 2007	Cattaneo et al,[49] 2012	D'Orio et al,[44] 2012	Cameron & Lord,[22] 2010	Matsuda et al,[41] 2012	Cameron et al,[45] 2011
Study focus	Accidental falls	Factors for falls	HCP response to falls	Injurious falls	Falls risk in MS	Falls using AD	Perceived fall risk	Falls in women	Factors for falls	Lesion site and falls	FoF falls	VTC in MS vs HS	Cognition and falls	Postural control	FoF & reasons for falls	Falls with injury
Balance deficits & postural control	(+)	(+)	(+)	(+)	(+)	(−)	(+)	(+)	(+)	(+)	(+)	(+)		(+)		
Age	(−)	(−)	(−)	(−)	(+)	(−)		(−)	(−)	(−)	(−)		(−)			
Gender (F or M)	(−)	(+M)	(−)	(−)		(−)			(−)	(−)	(+F)	(−)	(−)			(+F)
Walking ability	(+)		(−)	(+)	(+)	(−)	(+)	(+)	(+)	(−)	(+)		(+)			
MS status (stable vs deteriorating)	(+)	(+)	(−)	(+)	(+)	(−)	(+)	(+)		(+)	(+)	(−)				
Use of assisted device	(+)		(+)	(−)	(+)		(−)		(+)		(+)	(−)				
Cognition	(−)	(+)	(+)				(+)		(−)		(+)		(+)			
FoF	(−)	(+)	(+)	(+)	(−)	(−)	(+)								(+)	
Weakness/Fatigue	(−)	(+)	(+)		(+)	(+)	(+)	(+)								
Spasticity	(+)	(+)	(+)	(+)	(+)											
Proprioception	(+)	(+)	(+)	(+)		(−)	(+)						(+)			
Bladder incontinence	(−)	(+)	(−)	(+)		(−)										

Abbreviations: F, female; FoF, fear of falling; HCP, health care provider; M, male; MS, multiple sclerosis.

reduced both the number of fallers and the number of falls. Further study for treatment and intervention is warranted because of the high number of falls reported in this population.

Common outcome measures in multiple sclerosis for ambulation and balance

Walking and balance limitations are some of the most visible and common manifestations of impairment in MS.[51] Regular assessment of balance and walking with reliable and valid outcome measures helps direct patient care and intervention. The following sections describe common outcome measures used by physical therapists in the clinical setting to evaluate gait and balance.

Walking measures

12-item multiple sclerosis walking scale The 12-item MS walking scale (MSWS-12) is a self-report measure of the impact of motor fatigue on walking.[52] Nilsagard and colleagues[37] found a cutoff score of 75 had a sensitivity of 52% and a specificity of 82% in predicting fallers versus nonfallers in 76 patients with MS; EDSS were scores 3.5 to 6.0. This study also found a test-retest intraclass correlation coefficient (ICC) of 0.94.

EDSS The EDSS is a 0- to 10-point scale in which walking is measured in the middle range from 4.5 to 7.5 using need for assistive device and maximum distance walked up to 500 m as measures. The EDSS is useful for assessing disease severity; however, it is only marginally useful in assessing walking performance because many researchers have found a bimodal frequency distribution in which the middle ranges are not as well represented.[53] Historically, the EDSS demonstrates poor psychometric properties with low sensitivity, poor reliability, and low responsiveness to change.[51]

Hauser ambulation index The Hauser ambulation index (HAI) is a 10-point scale (0 = no impairment to 9 = confinement to wheelchair) dependent on need for an assistive device and the time to walk 25 feet. In one study by Cattaneo and colleagues,[54] the HAI was not able to distinguish between fallers and nonfallers. This scale has demonstrated high inter-rater and intra-rater reliability at ICC of 0.96 and 0.93, respectively, but has demonstrated low responsiveness to change with an effect size of 0.2.[53]

Modified functional walking categories The modified functional walking categories (MFWC) is a categorical scale from 1 (physiologic walker) to 6 (unlimited community walker) that focuses on the skills necessary for home and community ambulation, including the ability to negotiate curbs, crowded environments, stairs, and uneven terrain in the community. It also addresses levels of supervision needed for walking within and outside of the home and home mobility with and without a wheelchair. In a 2011 study by Kempen and colleagues,[55] a specific cutoff gait speed was found for each level of community walking on the MFWC using 10-minute walk test (10MWT) (unlimited community walker [cw] = 1.63 m/s, least-limited cw = 1.35 m/s, most-limited cw = 1.04 m/s, unlimited household walker = .48 m/s).

6MWT and 2MWT In a study by Goldman and colleagues,[56] the 6MWT demonstrated excellent intra-rater ICC of 0.95 and inter-rater reliability with an ICC of 0.91 in 40 patients with EDSS of 0 to 6.5 (20 controls). Patients with MS demonstrated reduced 6MWT distances compared with controls and 6MWT distance was reduced with increasing disability. Learmonth and colleagues[57] established the minimal detectable change (MDC) to be 76.2 m with a standard error of measurement (SEM) to be 27.48 m. In a study by Wetzel and colleagues,[58] 6MWT performance was found to differ significantly between patients with MS with mild (EDSS <4 = 402.4 m) and moderate (EDSS 4.0–6.5 = 193.7 m) disability. They found that decreased balance confidence and lower extremity power were correlated with increased risk for disability, as patients with MS were not able to reach the 350-m threshold required for even a single-task community ambulation. Because of the possible constraints on patients with MS due to fatigue, the 2MWT test may be more feasible than the 6MWT in patients with MS.[51] However, the reliability of the 2MWT has not yet been reported.[52]

Six-spot step test In the 6-spot step test (6SST), the patient is instructed to walk as fast as possible while kicking blocks out of marked circles with the same foot alternating between using the medial and lateral side of the foot around a rectangular field 1 m wide × 5 m in length. The 6SST is scored by calculating the mean time of 4 runs (2 runs with each foot). The 6SST demonstrated excellent test-retest reliability with an ICC of 0.95 and was strongly correlated with the Timed 25-ft Walk (T25FW) with a Spearman's r of 0.80.[59]

Gait speed measures

10MWT The 10MWT has demonstrated excellent reproducibility in a study with an ICC of 0.92 with the smallest percentage difference needed to detect genuine change of −23% or +30% change in time for the 10MWT.[60] There is little consensus among studies on what constitutes a minimally important clinical difference (MICD), with some studies showing an increase of 0.17 m/s or a decrease of 0.12 m/s,[61] or a change of 0.26 m/s in speed[62] verses a change in time of 28%[63] as meaningful. One study reported a strong correlation of $r = 0.95$ when comparing maximal speed of the 10MWT and the 6MWT.[64]

Timed 25-foot walk In patients with MS and EDSS 5.0 to 6.5, Learmonth and colleagues[57] found the reliability of the timed 25-foot walk (T25FW) to be ICC of 0.94 with an MCD of 12.6 seconds and the standard error of measurement to be 4.56 seconds. Multiple studies report a more than 20% change in time on the T25FW as a clinically meaningful difference in gait speed.[52]

30MWT The 30MWT has demonstrated excellent reproducibility with ICC of 0.93. The smallest percentage difference needed to detect genuine change varies with disability status (−14% to +17% change in time in those with EDSS ≤4 vs −38% to +60% for EDSS >4), with those with less disability demonstrating smaller performance changes for meaningful differences.[60]

Balance measures

Activities-specific balance confidence The activities-specific balance confidence (ABC) scale is a 16-item self-report measure in which patients rate their percent of balance confidence (0%–100%) in performing several functional activities. It was validated in people with mild to moderate MS with high ICC of 95 and was able to distinguish multiple fallers from nonfallers, but not from single fallers.[65] Cattaneo and colleagues[66] also validated the ABC's test-retest reliability at 0.92 with the standard error of measurement of 7.14. In another study by Cattaneo and colleagues,[54] a score of 40% was identified as a cutoff for risk of falls with a sensitivity of 65% and specificity of 77%.

Balance evaluation systems test This clinical balance assessment tool of 36 items examines different functional balance control systems for a comprehensive balance evaluation. In a small study (n of 13 patients with MS and 13 healthy controls) by Jacobs and Kasser,[67] subjects with MS exhibited significantly lower scores on the balance evaluation system test (BESTest) than controls, which also correlated with peak

CoP displacements on leaning and postural response tasks and step velocity during step initiation but not to anticipatory postural reactions. The regression models demonstrated that the BESTest can provide 86% of the sensitivity to identify fallers and 95% of the specificity to identify nonfallers.

Berg balance scale The Berg balance scale (BBS) is a classic balance outcome measure composed of 14 items designed to assess static balance and fall risk. In patients with MS EDSS of 5.0 to 6.5, Learmonth and colleagues[57] found the reliability of the BBS to be ICC of 0.96 with an MCD of 7 points and the standard error of measurement to be 3 points. In one study by Cattaneo and colleagues,[66] the inter-rater reliability was 0.96 with test-retest reliability at 0.96 with the standard error of measurement ranging between 1.48 and 1.51. In another study by Cattaneo and colleagues,[54] a score of 44 was identified as a cutoff for risk of falls with poor sensitivity of 40% but good specificity of 90%, indicating the BBS better identifies nonfallers correctly.

Dizziness handicap inventory The dizziness handicap inventory (DHI) is a 25-item self-assessment designed to evaluate the self-perceived effects of dizziness on daily function. In one study by Cattaneo and colleagues,[66] test-retest reliability was found with an ICC of 0.90. In another study by Cattaneo and colleagues,[54] a score of less than 59 was identified as a cutoff for risk of falls with a sensitivity of 50% and specificity of 74%.

Dynamic gait index The dynamic gait index (DGI) is an 8-item ambulation assessment to measure dynamic balance. The DGI has demonstrated good inter-rater reliability with an ICC of 0.98 and intra-rater reliability from 0.76 to 0.98 in patients with MS EDSS of 2.0 to 6.0.[68] In another study, inter-rater reliability was 0.94 with test-retest reliability at 0.85.[66] In 2006, Cattaneo and colleagues,[54] also found that a score less than 12 was the cutoff for risk of falls with poor sensitivity of 45% but moderate to good specificity of 80%, indicating the DGI identifies nonfallers better than fallers.

Timed up and go The timed up and go (TUG) is a short test designed to assess walking, transfers, and fall risk. In patients with MS EDSS of 5.0 to 6.5, Learmonth and colleagues[57] found the reliability of the TUG to be ICC of 0.97 with an MCD of 10.6 seconds and the standard error of measurement to be 3.81 seconds. Similar findings were reported by Nilsagard and colleagues,[60] with an ICC of 0.91 for test-retest reliability. The smallest percentage difference needed to detect genuine change was approximately a −24% or +31% change in time for the TUG. However, in a study by Cattaneo and colleagues, no cutoff scores were established for falls, as the TUG was not able to discriminate between fallers and nonfallers.

INTERVENTION/TREATMENTS
Locomotor Training

Locomotor training is a task-oriented intervention aimed at improving walking ability in individuals who have experienced neurologic injuries, such as spinal cord injury or stroke.[69] Two types of locomotor training have emerged, including body weight support treadmill training (BWSTT) and robotic-assisted treadmill training (RAGT). Both involve suspending the patient in a harness over a treadmill to assist with unweighting a percentage of body weight. The BWSTT intervention can require 1 to 3 therapists or aids who facilitate a normal walking pattern by providing manual assistance on key landmarks during each part of the gait cycle. Harkema and colleagues[70] developed principles to improve the efficiency of intervention by providing sensory input consistent with normal walking and encouraging trunk, limb, and pelvic kinematics to decrease compensatory strategies and promote upright control. During RAGT, a motorized, robotically driven gait orthosis moves the patient's lower extremities through the gait cycle. RAGT is purported to decrease effort for the physical therapist, facilitate longer session duration, create kinematically correct and reproducible gait patterns, and improve measurement of patient performance.[71] Both of these methods have been researched in a variety of neurologic populations, and results are generally compared with conventional over-ground walking training (COGWT), but evidence is more limited in people with MS.

BWSTT has been reported to benefit patients with MS.[69,72] In 2005, Fulk[69] found BWSTT in patients with MS resulted in significant improvement in gait speed (10MWT), walking endurance (6MWT), and participation in daily social activities. Improvements were maintained at a 2-month follow-up. Fulk[69] was surprised that clients reported the cognitive demands of walking to be almost as challenging as the physical task itself. He suggested future research should explore the cognitive demands of BWSTT and its effect on outcomes. Giesser and colleagues[72] studied a small sample of 4 patients with secondary progressive MS (EDSS 7.0–7.5) who completed an average of 40 sessions of BWSTT. They found that 1 of 4 patients had a positive change in EDSS score.[72] All patients significantly improved gait speed and strength, whereas 3 of 4 patients showed improved endurance, decreased lower extremity tone, and increased quality of life.[72] Overall, their small study showed that patients with severely impaired ambulation due to MS can tolerate and benefit from BWSTT.[72]

Several studies to date have compared RAGT with either BWSTT or COGWT.[71,73–76] Lo and Triche[71] studied outcomes in a crossover study starting either with BWSTT then moving to RAGT following a wash-out period. Thirteen patients with MS (EDSS mean of 4.9) participated in 3 weeks of each intervention with no statistically significant difference between groups, but significant improvement in primary gait outcomes, such as the T25FW, the 6MWT, percentage of double stance time, and the EDSS score. Wier and colleagues[73] studied quality of life in the same study, with participants demonstrating no significant difference between RAGT and BWSTT for improving quality of life in the crossover design.

Vaney and colleagues[74] compared RAGT to COGWT in 49 patients with MS (EDSS 3.0–6.5) with each group receiving 9 sessions. They measured quality of life, walking speed, and energy expenditure between groups. No statistically significant difference was found in any of the outcome measures; however, between-group difference was in favor of the COGWT group with regard to gait speed (by 0.08 m/s) and quality of life.[74] In contrast, Beer and colleagues[75] studied 35 patients with MS with slightly higher EDSS (6.0–7.5) completing 15 sessions of RAGT versus COGWT. Results demonstrated a moderate to large effect size (0.7) in gait speed, walking distance, and the knee extensors in these measures in the RAGT group, whereas the COGWT group had a significant improvement only in gait speed. Both groups returned to baseline at follow-up 6 months postintervention.[75]

A prospective randomized controlled trial by Schwartz and colleagues[76] compared RAGT with COGWT in 32 patients with MS (EDSS 5–7) participating in 12 sessions. Transient significant changes were found in 6MWT, 10MWT, BBS, and TUG following treatment and 3 months posttreatment between groups; however, none of the changes were retained at 6 months. Overall, there is limited research on locomotor training in patients with MS. There is a mild trend showing a positive immediate benefit, but limited carryover and no significant difference between RAGT or BWSTT. Further investigation in this subject is required.

Functional Electrical Stimulation

Functional electrical stimulation (FES) is a clinical application of a small electrical current to trigger a muscle contraction that is then incorporated into a functional activity. Electricity applied across the surface of the skin on an intact peripheral nerve fiber causes the muscle to contract. This stimulation is used to stimulate the muscles that lift the foot during the swing phase of gait.[77]

Patients with MS frequently have trouble with drop foot because of inadequate strength in the dorsiflexors. This weakness causes patients to catch their foot while taking a step, putting them at an increased fall risk. Liberson and colleagues[78] introduced the first drop foot stimulator in 1961. FES can be used with a heel switch to activate the dorsiflexors at the appropriate time in the gait cycle to help clear the foot.[79]

Numerous studies have demonstrated the effectiveness of FES in treating foot drop in patients with MS. Carnstam and colleagues[80] reported an increase in dorsiflexor strength and a reduction of calf tone after 10 to 15 minutes of stimulation when working with patients with MS. Karnia and colleagues[81] looked at 43 patients with MS; after 18 weeks of stimulation, 21 subjects demonstrated a mean increase of 16% in walking speed and a reduction in energy expenditure by 24%. Taylor and colleagues,[82] in another study of 78 subjects, showed improvement in unassisted walking speed of more than 10% with use of FES.

The literature also shows that for longer-term strengthening of the dorsiflexors, a simple program of home exercise delivers a more effective means of improving unassisted walking performance for patients with MS than by the use of FES alone.[79] Evidence supports the efficacy of an orthotic effect when using FES during both short distance and endurance walking in patients with MS with increased disability. However, in the same study, FES use in less disabled patients with MS was not shown to increase the speed of short distance walking.[83]

FES devices have been geared toward assisting with foot drop through stimulation of the common fibular nerve. There are many products on the market to assist with toe clearance, including the Bioness L300 foot drop system, Walkaide, and the Odstock dropped foot stimulator. There are also some new products available that help with knee stability that stimulate the quadriceps as well, such as the Bioness L300 Plus and the Odstock 2-channel stimulator.

There are contraindications to using FES (eg, patients who have a pacemaker, lower motor neuron nerve injury, and skin sensitivity), so this treatment must be prescribed by a physician.[14] There are limitations of FES when compared with an ankle foot orthosis. FES does not provide any medial-lateral stability, it is costly, takes more effort to use, and does not work for everyone.

An FES bike that allows the equivalent of 300 steps in 1 hour is available in many clinics. This bike allows for synchronized firing of the muscles used for cycling. A pilot study by Ratchford and colleagues[84] looked at FES cycling with patients with MS and found that it was reasonably well tolerated, and encouraging improvements were seen in walking and quality of life measures.

Medications to Improve Gait

Compounded 4-amino pyridine (4AP) has been use for decades to improve ambulation and function in MS. However, the window between efficacy and toxicity (most common adverse event is seizures) is very narrow and, as the compound is metabolized relatively quickly, it had always been difficult to maintain a safe therapeutic level. This problem has recently been resolved, and a new, sustained-release formulation has become available. Dalfampridine (Ampyra) has been approved by the FDA to improve walking in MS. Clinical trials indicated that there were "responders" and "non-responders"; approximately 40% of subjects were responders. It comes in a 10-mg coated tablet, and is taken every 12 hours.[85–87]

Orthotics

Lower-extremity braces or ankle foot orthoses (AFOs) are used to improve deficits in gait and to promote safe ambulation in patients with central neurologic disorders such as MS.[14,48,88–91] AFOs can be used to address problems including decreased foot clearance in the swing phase of gait, reduced heel strike at initial contact, and poor stability in the stance phase.[14,48,88–90] AFOs are effective for compensating for weakness, restoring energy, and ankle/knee control.[14] A variety of braces are available for different types of gait deficits (**Table 2**) providing varying support throughout the gait cycle. AFOs can be made of lightweight plastic, metal, or carbon fiber. Knee/ankle/foot orthoses (KAFOs) are rarely recommended for patients with MS because of the increased energy cost and added weight to the weak limb during ambulation.[14,97]

AFOs are also recommended for balance and decreased energy cost of walking. Cattaneo and colleagues[48] found that static (solid ankle) and dynamic (hinged and flexible) AFOs improve static balance, but not dynamic balance in patients with MS. Ramdharry and colleagues[89] looked at the use of dynamic foot orthoses (DFOs), an orthosis contoured to correspond to the dynamic arches of the foot, on balance and walking. They found that although DFOs initially seemed to cause an increase in postural sway, over a 4-week period, patients demonstrated an apparent training effect with a reduction in sway when eyes were closed and a subjective report of improved walking and balance function. Perry and colleagues[90] found that the use of a rocker shoe as a walking aid in selected patients with MS showed a decrease in the net energy cost of ambulation. Bregman and colleagues[95,96] studied the effect of AFOs on the cost of energy during walking and found that the energy requirements may be decreased by choosing an AFO that has the proper amount of stiffness and energy storage. Although an AFO can be effective for some patients with MS, it can have poor, or even adverse effects, in others.[88,95,96] Patient-specific prescriptions of the proper AFOs are essential and can be recommended by a physical therapist and/or an orthotist.[93]

Assistive Devices

Single-point canes enlarge a patient's base of support (BoS) and are recommended to assist with even weight distribution during ambulation. They function best for patients with mildly unstable gait and moderate balance control. Quad canes provide a little more stability over uneven surfaces, but tend to decrease overall gait velocity and do not improve asymmetrical gait patterns.[98] Forearm crutches provide a larger BoS than a cane, help decrease weight bearing on a single lower extremity, and are recommended for patients with good upper extremity control and mild to moderate balance deficits. Walkers provide the largest base of stability for increased stability during ambulation and come in a variety of options. Walkers are usually recommended for patients with MS with moderate gait and balance deficits.

Referral to physical therapy for assistive device prescription is important to ensure the patient has the most appropriate device for his or her current level of function and lifestyle.[97]

Wheelchair Mobility

Because of weakness, decreased balance, spasticity, and fatigue, many patients with MS must use a wheelchair as their only safe option for independent mobility.[14,97]

Table 2
Bracing recommendations for patients with multiple sclerosis

Deficit/Limitation	Gait Impairment[7,92]	Potentially Beneficial Orthosis[93]
Hip control		
Hip flexor weakness	↓ LE clearance in swing phase, toe drag Weak limb circumduction Contralateral lean of the trunk Contralateral vaulting to clear weak leg Shortened stride length	Hip flexion assist orthosis[94]
Hip extensor weakness	Forward trunk lean in swing Backward lean in stance for compensation	None
Knee control		
Quad spasticity (knee extension)	↑ Knee extension in stance phase	AFO with PF stop (↑ toe clearance)
Hamstring spasticity (knee flexion)	Crouched gait pattern ↑ Knee flexion at IC and during stance ↑ Demand on quads for stability Shortened stride length	Ground Reaction Force AFO Carbon fiber AFO Articulated AFO with PF/DF stop (↓ toe clearance)
Quad weakness	↓ Control of knee flexion in mid stance Knee hyperextension at IC Forward trunk lean compensation	Articulated AFO with DF stop (↓ tibial translation) Ground reaction force AFO
Hamstring weakness	Knee hyperextension in mid to late stance due to ↓ ability to slow limb	Articulated AFO with PF stop (↑ toe clearance)
Ankle control		
DF weakness	Foot drop, inability to clear toes ↑ Hip/knee flexion during swing phase Circumduction/lateral lean for ↑ LE clearance	Posterior leaf spring AFO[88,95,96] Articulated AFO with DF/PF stop
PF weakness	Knee hyperextension in mid-late stance phase ↓ Push off during preswing	Posterior leaf spring AFO[88,95,96] Carbon fiber AFO[88,95,96] Articulated AFO with PF stop
DF Spasticity	↑ Ankle inversion if tibialis anterior implicated	Articulated AFO with DF stop
PF Spasticity	↑ Knee hyperextension during stance and ↓ push off	Articulated AFO with PF stop Solid ankle AFO for ↓ stretch reflex[97]
Mediolateral instability	Inversion/eversion during stance Instability in stance Possible toe drag during swing	Solid ankle AFO[14,97] Articulated AFO[14,97] Double metal upright (same)

Abbreviations: AFO, ankle foot orthosis; DF, dorsiflexion; IC, initial contact in gait cycle; LE, lower extremity; PF, plantarflexion.

There are many options for manual and powered mobility. If upper extremity strength is adequate to push a wheelchair, a variety of lightweight manual wheelchairs are available. A patient will need to consider rigid versus folding options. A rigid frame provides more efficient propulsion because no energy is lost in the cross frame, as with a folding wheelchair.[14] Rigid frame chairs offer the greatest amount of seat adjustment, allowing for optimal posture and stability. The weight of the chair must also be considered. Great advancements have been made in bringing the overall weight of the chair down, which is critical for a population with strength and endurance issues.[14] Different accessories, such as plastic-coated hand rims for someone with decreased hand function can make wheelchair propulsion easier. It is important to consider the patient's shoulder integrity, cardiovascular endurance, and coordination when deciding between power and manual wheelchair use.[14,97] New products are available on the market that can be installed on a manual wheelchair to provide power-assisted propulsion (eg, Smart Drive, Magic Wheels, and Widgit), which increase the effectiveness of the push.[14] Wheelchair transportation must also be considered. Folding manual chairs allow for quick, easy stowage, whereas power wheelchairs can generally not be transported in a car and require a lift or wheelchair-accessible van.

Powered mobility allows patients to conserve their energy for other important daily tasks.[14,97] A common strategy is to use a wheelchair for covering longer distances, and walking to cover shorter distances. If a patient has trunk control and good sitting balance, powered scooters may be an option. The scooter seat swivels, allowing patients to get closer to transferring surfaces. Scooters can also be broken down for transport in a car. A power wheelchair with a tilt system is used when patients' weakness or tone does not allow them to change their position in their chair.[14] They require this tilt system to get pressure off of their weight-bearing surfaces to avoid skin breakdown and decubitus ulcers.[14] If the patient has decreased sensation, a proper pressure-relieving cushion must also be prescribed to reduce the risk of pressure sores.[14]

Power wheelchairs can be operated by the hand, foot, chin, head, mouth, eye gaze systems, or proximity switches. It is critical that a power-wheelchair user have adequate vision, judgment, and cognition to drive the chair safely and not be at risk for injuring either oneself or others while driving.[14,97] To drive a wheelchair successfully, proper positioning needs to be addressed. If patients do not have adequate head and trunk support, they will not be able to use their available upper extremity strength to the greatest capability.[14] Trunk supports, hip guides, and angled seats/backs/headrests can be added and modified to maximize available function. When prescribing a wheelchair for a patient with MS, it is important to order a wheelchair that can accommodate necessary modifications if the disease progresses and function declines. A physical therapist should be consulted to train patients in advanced wheelchair skills, which can greatly improve function in the community.

SUMMARY

MS is an immune-mediated disease that causes demyelination and neural degeneration within the CNS. The pathology results in many impairments, including muscle weakness, abnormal tone, visual disturbances, decreased sensation, and fatigue. Rehabilitation helps patients with MS maximize independence by helping to manage and minimize impairments; early referral to physical therapy is a must. Deficits seen in ambulation should be addressed to improve energy efficiency and reduce falls. Compensation through appropriate prescription of assistive devices, bracing, and wheelchairs will help improve safety. Rehabilitation can make a significant impact on achieving and maintaining quality of life and independence.

REFERENCES

1. Kraft GH. Prevalence and diagnosis of walking impairments in patients with multiple sclerosis. Neurol Rev, in press.
2. Goodman AD, Brown TR, Krupp LB, et al. Sustained-release oral fampridine in multiple sclerosis: a randomized, double-blind, controlled trial. Lancet 2009; 373(9665):732–8.
3. Kraft GH. Rehabilitation still the only way to improve function in multiple sclerosis. Lancet 1999;354(9195):2016–7.
4. Cameron MH, Wagner JM. Gait abnormalities in multiple sclerosis: pathogenesis, evaluation, and advances in treatment. Curr Neurol Neurosci Rep 2011;11:507–15.
5. Kurtzke JF. Rating neurologic impairment in multiple sclerosis: an expanded disability status scale (EDSS). Neurology 1983;33(11):1444–52.
6. Sosnoff JJ, Sandroff BM, Motl RW. Quantifying gait abnormalities in persons with multiple sclerosis with minimal disability. Gait Posture 2012;36:154–6.
7. Shumway-Cook A, Woollacott MH. Motor control: translating research into clinical practice. 3rd edition. Philadelphia: Lippincott Williams & Wilkins; 2007.
8. Kraft GH, Alquist AD, de Lateur BJ. Effect of microclimate cooling on physical function in multiple sclerosis. Multiple Sclerosis Clinical and Laboratory Research 1996;2(2):114–5.
9. Robinson LR, Kraft GH, Fitts SS, et al. Body cooling may not improve somatosensory pathway function in multiple sclerosis. Am J Phys Med Rehabil 1997; 76(3):191–6.
10. Guitierrez G, Chow JW, Tillman MD, et al. Resistance training improves gait kinematics in persons with MS. Arch Phys Med Rehabil 2005;86(9):1824–9.
11. Kraft GH, Alquist AD, Lateur BJ. Effects of resistive exercise on function in multiple sclerosis (MS). Arch Phys Med Rehabil 1996;77:984.
12. DeBolt LS, McCubbin JA. The effects of home-based resistance exercise on power, balance and mobility in adults with MS. Arch Phys Med Rehabil 2004;85: 290–7.
13. Barnes MP, Kent RM, Semlyen JK, et al. Spasticity in multiple sclerosis. Neurorehabil Neural Repair 2003;17:66–70.
14. O'Sullivan SB, Schmitz TJ. Physical rehabilitation. 5th edition. Philadelphia: F.A. Davis Co; 2007.
15. Freal JE, Kraft GH, Coryell JK. Symptomatic fatigue in multiple sclerosis. Arch Phys Med Rehabil 1984;65(3):135–8.
16. Kraft GH, Freal JE, Coryell JK. Disability, disease duration, and rehabilitation service needs in multiple sclerosis: patient perspectives. Arch Phys Med Rehabil 1986;67(3):164–8.
17. Herndon RM, Horak F. Vertigo, imbalance, and incoordination. In: Burks JS, Johnson KP, editors. Multiple sclerosis: diagnosis, medical management and rehabilitation. New York: Demos Medical Publishing; 2000. p. 333–9.
18. Cattaneo D, Jonsdottir J. Sensory impairments in quiet standing in subjects with multiple sclerosis. Mult Scler 2009;15:59–67.
19. Lundy-Eckman L. Neuroscience: fundamentals for rehabilitation. 3rd edition. St Louis (MO): Saunders Elsevier; 2007.
20. Pavan K, Marangoni BE, Schmidt KB, et al. Vestibular rehabilitation in patients with relapsing-remitting multiple sclerosis. Arq Neuropsiquiatr 2007;65(2A): 332–5 [in Portuguese].
21. Badke MB, Shea TA, Miedaner JA, et al. Outcomes after rehabilitation for adults with balance dysfunction. Arch Phys Med Rehabil 2004;85(2):227–33.

22. Cameron MH, Lord S. Postural control in multiple sclerosis: implications for fall prevention. Curr Neurol Neurosci Rep 2010;10:407–12.
23. Krishnan V, Kanekar N, Aruin AS. Feedforward postural control in individuals with multiple sclerosis during load release. Gait Posture 2012;36(2):225–30.
24. Boesa MK, Sosnoff JJ, Socie MJ, et al. Postural control in multiple sclerosis: effects of disability status and dual task. J Neurol Sci 2012;315:44–8.
25. Cattaneo D, Jonsdottir J, Zocchi M, et al. Effects of balance exercises on people with multiple sclerosis: a pilot study. Clin Rehabil 2007;21:771–81.
26. Zeigelboim B, Liberalesso P, Jurkiewicz A, et al. Clinical benefits to vestibular rehabilitation in multiple sclerosis: a report of 4 cases. Int Tinnitus J 2010; 16(1):60–5.
27. Herbert JR, Corboy JR, Manago MM, et al. Effects of vestibular rehabilitation on multiple sclerosis-related fatigue and upright postural control: a randomised controlled trial. Phys Ther 2011;91(8):1166–83.
28. Freeman JA, Gear M, Pauli A, et al. The effect of core stability training on balance and mobility in ambulant individuals with multiple sclerosis: a multi-centre series of single case studies. Mult Scler 2010;16(11):1377–84.
29. Muñoz-Lasal S, Ferriero G, Valero R, et al. Effect of therapeutic horseback riding on balance and gait of people with multiple sclerosis. G Ital Med Lav Ergon 2011;33(4):462–7.
30. Bronson C, Brewerton K, Ong J, et al. Does hippotherapy improve balance in persons with multiple sclerosis: a systematic review. Eur J Phys Rehabil Med 2010;46(3):347–53.
31. Nilsagård YE, Forsberg AS, von Koch L. Balance exercise for persons with multiple sclerosis using Wii games: a randomised, controlled multi-centre study. Mult Scler 2012;19(2):1–8.
32. Widener GL, Allen DD, Gibson-Horn C. Randomized clinical trial of balance-based torso weighting for improving upright mobility in people with multiple sclerosis. Neurorehabil Neural Repair 2009;23(8):784–91.
33. Gibson-Horn C. Balance-based torso-weighting in a patient with ataxia and multiple sclerosis: a case report. J Neurol Phys Ther 2008;32(3):139–46.
34. Finlayson ML, Peterson E, Cho CC. Risk factors for falling among people aged 45 to 90 years with multiple sclerosis. Arch Phys Med Rehabil 2006;87:1274–9.
35. Peterson EW, Cho CC, Von Koch L, et al. Injurious falls among middle aged and older adults with multiple sclerosis. Arch Phys Med Rehabil 2008;89:1031–7.
36. Peterson EW, Cho CC, Finlayson ML. Fear of falling and associated activity curtailment among middle aged and older adults with multiple sclerosis. Mult Scler 2007;13:1168–75.
37. Nilsagard Y, Lundholm C, Denison E, et al. Predicting accidental falls in people with multiple sclerosis—a longitudinal study. Clin Rehabil 2009;23:259–69.
38. Kasser SL, Jacobs JV, Foley JT, et al. A prospective evaluation of balance, gait and strength to predict falling in women with multiple sclerosis. Arch Phys Med Rehabil 2011;92:1840–6.
39. Prosperini L, Kouleridou A, Petsas N, et al. The relationship between infratentorial lesions, balance deficit and accidental falls in multiple sclerosis. J Neurol Sci 2011;304:55–60.
40. Sosnoff JJ, Socie MJ, Boes MK, et al. Mobility, balance and falls in persons with multiple sclerosis. PLoS One 2011;6(11):e28021.
41. Matsuda PN, Shumway-Cook A, Ciol MA, et al. Understanding falls in multiple sclerosis: association of mobility status, concerns about falling, and accumulated impairments. Phys Ther 2012;92:407–15.

42. Matsuda PN, Shumway-Cook A, Bamer AM, et al. Falls in multiple sclerosis. PM R 2011;3:624–32.

43. Coote S, Hogan N, Franklin S. Falls in people with MS who use a walking aid: prevalence, factors and effect of balance and strengthening interventions. Arch Phys Med Rehabil 2012. http://dx.doi.org/10.1016/j.apmr.2012.10.020.

44. D'Orio VL, Foley FW, Armentano F, et al. Cognitive and motor functioning in patients with multiple sclerosis: neuropsychological predictors of walking speed and falls. J Neurol Sci 2012;316:42–6.

45. Cameron MH, Poel AJ, Haselkorn JK, et al. Falls requiring medical attention among veterans with multiple sclerosis: a cohort study. J Rehabil Res Dev 2011;48(1):13–20.

46. Nilsagard Y, Denison E, Gunnarsson LG, et al. Factors perceived as being related to accidental falls by persons with multiple sclerosis. Disabil Rehabil 2009;31:1301–10.

47. Cattaneo D, De Nuzzo C, Fascia T, et al. Risks of falls in subjects with multiple sclerosis. Arch Phys Med Rehabil 2002;83:864–7.

48. Cattaneo D, Marazzini F, Crippa A, et al. Do static or dynamic AFOs improve balance? Clin Rehabil 2002;16:894–9.

49. Cattaneo D, Ferrarin M, Jonsdottir J, et al. The virtual time to contact in the evaluation of balance disorders and prediction of falls in people with multiple sclerosis. Disabil Rehabil 2012;34:470–7.

50. Finlayson M, Peterson EW, Cho C. Pilot study of a fall risk management program for middle aged and older adults with MS. NeuroRehabilitation 2009;25:107–15.

51. Bethoux F, Bennett S. Evaluating walking in patients with multiple sclerosis: which assessment tools are useful in clinical practice? Int J MS Care 2011;13: 4–14.

52. Kieseier BC, Pozzilli C. Assessing walking disability in multiple sclerosis. Mult Scler 2012;18(7):914–24.

53. Sharrack B, Hughes RA, Soudain S, et al. The psychometric properties of clinical rating scales used in multiple sclerosis. Brain 1999;122:141–59.

54. Cattaneo D, Regola A, Meotti M. Validity of six balance disorder scales in persons with multiple sclerosis. Disabil Rehabil 2006;28(12):789–95.

55. Kempen JC, de Groot V, Knol DL, et al. Community walking can be assessed using a 10-metre timed walk test. Mult Scler 2011;17(8):980–90.

56. Goldman M, Marrie RA, Cohen JA. Evaluation of the six-minute walk in multiple sclerosis subjects and healthy controls. Mult Scler 2007;14:383–90.

57. Learmonth YC, Paul L, McFadyen AK, et al. Reliability and clinical significance of mobility and balance assessments in multiple sclerosis. Int J Rehabil Res 2012;35(1):69–74.

58. Wetzel JL, Fry DK, Pfalzer LA. Six-minute walk test for persons with mild or moderate disability from multiple sclerosis: performance and explanatory factors. Physiother Can 2010;63(2):166–80.

59. Nieuwenhuis MM, Van Tongeren H, Sorensen PS, et al. The six spot step test: a new measurement for walking ability in multiple sclerosis. Mult Scler 2006;12: 495–500.

60. Nilsagard Y, Lundholm C, Gunnarsson LG, et al. Clinical relevance using timed walk tests and 'timed up and go' testing in persons with multiple sclerosis. Physiother Res Int 2007;12(2):105–14.

61. Morris ME, Cantwell C, Vowels L, et al. Changes in gait and fatigue from morning to afternoon in people with multiple sclerosis. J Neurol Neurosurg Psychiatry 2002;72:361–5.

62. Paltamaa J, Sarasoja T, Leskinen E, et al. Measuring deterioration in international classification of functioning domains of people with multiple sclerosis who are ambulatory. Phys Ther 2008;88:176–90.

63. Vaney C, Blaurock H, Gattlen B, et al. Assessing mobility in multiple sclerosis using the Rivermead Mobility Index and gait speed. Clin Rehabil 1996;10: 216–26.

64. Dalgas U, Severinsen K, Overgaard K. Relations between 6 minute walking distance and 10 meter walking speed in patients with multiple sclerosis and stroke. Arch Phys Med Rehabil 2012;93:1167–72.

65. Nilsagard Y, Carling A, Forsberg A. Activities-specific balance confidence in people with multiple sclerosis. Mult Scler Int 2012;1–8. http://dx.doi.org/10. 1155/2012/613925.

66. Cattaneo D, Jonsdottir J, Repetti S. Reliability of four scales on balance disorders in persons with multiple sclerosis. Disabil Rehabil 2007;29(24):1920–5.

67. Jacobs JV, Kasser SL. Balance impairment in people with multiple sclerosis: preliminary evidence for the balance evaluation systems test. Gait Posture 2012;36:414–8.

68. McConvery J, Bennett SE. Reliability of the dynamic gait index in individuals with multiple sclerosis. Arch Phys Med Rehabil 2005;86:130–3.

69. Fulk GD. Locomotor training and virtual reality-based balance training for an individual with multiple sclerosis: a case report. J Neurol Phys Ther 2005;29(1): 34–42.

70. Harkema S, Behrman A, Barbeau H. Locomotor training: principles and practice. New York: Oxford University Press; 2011.

71. Lo AC, Triche EW. Improving gait in multiple sclerosis using robot-assisted, body weight supported treadmill training. Neurorehabil Neural Repair 2008; 22(6):661–71.

72. Giesser B, Beres-Jones J, Budovitch A, et al. Locomotor training using body weight support on a treadmill improves mobility in persons with multiple sclerosis: a pilot study. Mult Scler 2007;13:224–31.

73. Wier LM, Hatcher MS, Triche EW, et al. Effect of robot-assisted versus conventional body-weight-supported treadmill training on quality of life for people with multiple sclerosis. J Rehabil Res Dev 2011;48(4):483–92.

74. Vaney C, Gattlen B, Lugon-Moulin V, et al. Robotic-assisted step training (lokomat) not superior to equal intensity of over-ground rehabilitation in patients with multiple sclerosis. Neurorehabil Neural Repair 2012;26:212–21.

75. Beer S, Aschbacher B, Manoglou D, et al. Robot-assisted gait training in multiple sclerosis: a pilot randomized trial. Mult Scler 2008;14:231–6.

76. Schwartz I, Sajin A, Moreh E, et al. Robot-assisted gait training in multiple sclerosis patients: a randomized trial. Mult Scler 2012;18(6):881–90.

77. Zackowski K. Functional electrical stimulation: implications for neurorehabilitation in MS. Presented at: 2nd International Symposium on Gait and Balance in Multiple Sclerosis: Interventions for Gait & Balance in MS. Portland (OR): 2012.

78. Liberson WT, Holmquest HJ, Scot D, et al. Functional electrotherapy stimulation of the peroneal nerve synchronized with the swing phase of the gait of hemiplegic patients. Arch Phys Med Rehabil 1961;42:101–5.

79. Barrett CL, Mann GE, Taylor PN, et al. A randomized trial to investigate the effects of functional electrical stimulation and therapeutic exercise on walking performance for people with multiple sclerosis. Mult Scler 2009;15(4):493–504.

80. Carnstam B, Larsson LE, Prevec TS. Improvement in gait following electrical stimulation. Scand J Rehabil Med 1977;9:7–13.

81. Karnia A, Dillner S, Ebefors I, et al. Why patients use or reject a peroneal stimulator. Adv Extern Control Hum Extrem 1990;10:251–60.
82. Taylor PN, Burridge JH, Dunkerley AL, et al. Clinical use of the ODFS: its effect on walking speed and effort of walking. Arch Phys Med Rehabil 1999;80: 1577–83.
83. Stevens P, Hunsaker RB. Recent findings regarding the efficacy of functional electric stimulation in patients with chronic hemiplegia and multiple sclerosis: a narrative literature review. J Prosthet Orthot 2010;22(3):166–71.
84. Ratchford JN, Shore W, Hammond ER, et al. A pilot study of functional electrical stimulation cycling in progressive multiple sclerosis. NeuroRehabilitation 2010; 27(2):121–8.
85. Egeberg MD, Oh CY, Bainbridge JL. Clinical overview of dalfampridine: an agent with a novel mechanism of action to help with gait disturbances. Clin Ther 2012;34:2185–94.
86. Cook SD. Handbook of multiple sclerosis. 4th edition. New York: Taylor & Francis Group; 2006.
87. Rawlins PK. Intrathecal baclofen therapy over 10 years. J Neurosci Nurs 2004; 36(6):322–7.
88. Bregman DJ, DeGroot V, Van Diggele P, et al. Polypropylene ankle foot orthoses to overcome drop-foot gait in central neurological patients: a mechanical and functional evaluation. Prosthet Orthot Int 2010;34(3):293–304.
89. Ramdharry GM, Marsden JF, Day BL. De-stabilizing and training effects of foot orthoses in multiple sclerosis. Mult Scler 2006;12:219–26.
90. Perry J, Gronley JK, Lunsford T. Rocker shoe as walking aid in MS I. Arch Phys Med Rehabil 1981;62:59.
91. Sheffler LR, Hennessey MT, Knutson JS, et al. Functional effect of an ankle foot orthosis on gait in multiple sclerosis. Am J Phys Med Rehabil 2007;87(1):26–32.
92. Observational gait analysis handbook. Downey (CA): Los Amigo Research and Education Institute, Inc; 2001.
93. Kott K. Orthoses for patients with neurological disorders—clinical decision making. In: Seymour R, editor. Prosthetics and orthotics: lower limb and spinal. Baltimore (MD): Lippincott Williams & Wilkins; 2002.
94. Sutliff MH, Naft JM, Stoug DK, et al. Efficacy and safety of a hip flexion assist orthosis in ambulatory multiple sclerosis patients. Arch Phys Med Rehabil 2008;89:1611–7.
95. Bregman DJ, Van der Krogta MM, DeGroot V, et al. The effect of ankle foot orthosis stiffness on the energy cost of walking: a simulation study. Clin Biomech 2011;26:955–61.
96. Bregman DJ, Harlaara J, Meskers CG, et al. Spring-like ankle foot orthoses reduce the energy cost of walking by taking over ankle work. Gait Posture 2012;35:148–53.
97. Haselkorn J, Leer SE, Hall JA. Mobility. In: Burks JS, Johnson KP, editors. Multiple sclerosis: diagnosis, medical management and rehabilitation. New York: Demos Medical Publishing; 2000. p. 323–32.
98. Beauchamp MK, Skrela M, Southmayd D, et al. Immediate effects of cane use on gait symmetry in individuals with subacute stroke. Physiother Can 2009;61: 154–60.

Spasticity Management in Multiple Sclerosis

Christina Hughes, MD[a],*, Ileana M. Howard, MD[b]

KEYWORDS

- Spasticity • Multiple sclerosis • Antispasticity • Chemodenervation
- Intrathecal baclofen

KEY POINTS

- Spasticity is a prevalent and potentially disabling symptom common in individuals with multiple sclerosis.
- Adequate evaluation and management of spasticity requires a careful assessment of the patient's history to determine functional impact of spasticity and potential exacerbating factors, and physical examination to determine the extent of the condition and culpable muscles.
- A host of options for spasticity management are available: therapeutic exercise, physical modalities, complementary/alternative medicine interventions, oral medications, chemo-denervation, and implantation of an intrathecal baclofen pump.
- Choice of treatment hinges on a combination of the extent of the symptoms, patient preference, and availability of services.

CASE STUDY EXAMPLES

In this discussion of the evaluation and management of spasticity in multiple sclerosis (MS), it will be helpful to begin with two clinical scenarios. The first is an example of a common initial presentation of spasticity. Patient A is a 40-year-old woman with a 7-year history of relapsing remitting MS. Her disease course has been stable since initiation of glatiramer acetate (Copaxone) several years ago. She has no other medical history and is not on other medication besides supplemental vitamins. Functionally she is a very active individual and uses no assistive devices. She presents with tripping and near falls, involving catching her right toe, which occur mostly in the evening or at the end of a long hike. Her goal is to remain active with her outdoor activities. She has never had a spasticity treatment regimen.

[a] Department of Physical Medicine and Inpatient Neuro Rehabilitation, Virginia Mason Medical Center, Mailstop: H4-469, 1100 9th Avenue, Seattle, WA 98111, USA; [b] Rehabilitation Care Services, Veteran Affairs Puget Sound Health Care System, 1660 South Columbian Way, Seattle, WA 98108, USA
* Corresponding author.
E-mail address: pmrdoc@mac.com

Phys Med Rehabil Clin N Am 24 (2013) 593–604
http://dx.doi.org/10.1016/j.pmr.2013.07.003
1047-9651/13/$ – see front matter © 2013 Elsevier Inc. All rights reserved.

The second case is an example of multifactorial spasticity. Patient B is a 50-year-old man with a 20-year history of primary progressive MS. His disease course has been a slow, steady decline and he has never been on a disease-modifying agent. He has multiple medical comorbidities including active coronary artery disease, hypertension, hyperlipidemia, nephrolithiasis, and neurogenic bladder with suprapubic catheter. Functionally he is quadriplegic, but for many years has "used" his lower extremity spasticity to briefly perform standing pivot transfers with assistance, but uses a power wheelchair for all other mobility. Recently he began to have nighttime adductor spasticity with persistent scissoring of his legs that is uncomfortable and is interfering with his sleep. His spasticity treatment regimen for the past 10 years has been baclofen 20 mg at night, diazepam 5 mg at night, positioning, and daily stretching. His goal is to improve comfort and positioning in bed, and minimize side effects of medication.

SPASTICITY IN MULTIPLE SCLEROSIS

Spasticity can manifest in any condition that has upper motor neuron (UMN) lesions, including MS. The prevalence of spasticity in MS can be as high as 80%, and can present clinically and functionally in a variety of ways. Clinically, spasticity can manifest as stiffness of a muscle, muscle cramping, clonus, or periodic muscle spasms (flexor and extensor). It can present as a focal area of muscle tightness in an extremity or as a more diffuse process involving the torso and multiple extremities. Spasticity can be mild and may not interfere with function; however, up to one-third of patients may experience moderate to severe spasticity that limits activities of daily living and is associated with negative implications for quality of life.[1–3]

Spasticity can be a highly variable symptom that can be worsened by various stimuli. In general, it is worsened by any noxious stimuli to the body, which could be as simple as a change in temperature or body position, or more complex, such as acute illness. Common conditions that may worsen spasticity include infection (most commonly of the urinary tract), wounds, and constipation.[3]

PATHOPHYSIOLOGY OF SPASTICITY

In the literature, the definition of spasticity is often that given by Lance in 1980, which states: "Spasticity is a motor disorder characterized by a velocity dependent increase in tonic stretch reflexes ("muscle tone") with exaggerated tendon jerks, resulting from hyperexcitability of the stretch reflex as one component of the upper motor neurone syndrome."[4] Spasticity can occur whenever there is a lesion in a UMN pathway. The UMN pathways are descending motor tracts that originate in the cortex or brainstem and directly or indirectly influence the excitability of the lower motor neuron or anterior horn cell. These pathways include the corticospinal (pyramidal) tract, medial reticulospinal tract, lateral vestibular tract, and dorsal reticulospinal tract.[5]

Damage to the central nervous system can interrupt the UMN pathways and can cause a constellation of symptoms called the UMN syndrome. The UMN syndrome consists of positive features such as spasticity and spontaneous spasms and negative features such as weakness and decreased fine-motor control, which together impair functional movement. The constellation of symptoms in the UMN syndrome is detailed in **Table 1**.[3,5]

INITIAL EVALUATION OF THE PATIENT WITH SPASTICITY
History

Initial evaluation of the patient presenting for management of spasticity should include a focused history and physical examination, an evaluation of the patient's perception

Table 1
Summary of symptoms and signs of upper motor neuron syndrome

Negative	Positive
Weakness	Flexor/extensor spasms
Reduced dexterity	Spasticity
Reduced speed of movement	Dystonia
Fatigability	Increased tone
Slowed movements	Clonus
	Hyperactive deep tendon reflexes
	Babinski sign

of functional limitations arising from spasticity, and the goals of care. This assessment should include a brief but clear history of the patient's primary neurologic diagnosis; current symptoms and complaints related to spasticity; prior treatments, including medications, therapies, injections, surgeries, or other interventions; and pertinent medical history, including medication history and anticoagulation status. Review of systems should evaluate for signs and symptoms suggesting possible contributory factors, such as infection or noxious stimuli including fever/chills, dysuria, voiding difficulties, skin wounds, constipation, or acute pain.

Physical Examination

Physical examination should include assessment of the joints involved and surrounding joints, and should include passive and active range of motion, strength, sensation, reflexes, and assessment of spasticity. Several tools are available for rating spasticity, the most common of which are the Modified Ashworth Scale (MAS) and Tardieu scale (**Tables 2** and **3**).

The provider should observe, when able, the patient's functional mobility and any affected activities of daily living to gain further information before formalizing a treatment plan. Consideration that some patients use spasticity to enhance functional mobility (stabilizing gait or transfers) must be considered, to avoid inadvertently decreasing function with spasticity treatment. Common functional measures that can be used are outlined in **Box 1**.

Table 2
Modified Ashworth Scale (MAS)

Score	
0	No increase in muscle tone
1	Slight increase in muscle tone, manifested by a catch and release or by minimal resistance at the end range of motion when the part is moved
1+	Slight increase in muscle tone, manifested by a catch, followed by minimal resistance throughout the remainder (less than half) of the range
2	More marked increase in muscle tone throughout most of the range, but affected part is easily moved
3	Considerable increase in muscle tone, passive movement is difficult
4	Affected part is rigid

Table 3	
Tardieu scale	
Velocities	
V1	As slow as possible, slower than the natural drop of the limb segment under gravity
V2	Speed of limb segment falling under gravity
V3	As fast as possible, faster than the rate of the natural drop of the limb segment under gravity
Scoring	
0	No resistance throughout the course of the passive movement
1	Slight resistance throughout the course of passive movement, no clear catch at a precise angle
2	Clear catch at a precise angle, interrupting the passive movement, followed by release
3	Fatigable clonus with less than 10 s when maintaining the pressure and appearing at the precise angle
4	Unfatigable clonus with more than 10 s when maintaining the pressure and appearing at a precise angle
5	Joint is immovable

CONSERVATIVE TREATMENT STRATEGIES FOR SPASTICITY MANAGEMENT

Nonpharmacologic and noninvasive treatment interventions for spasticity provide primary or adjunctive intervention options to the individual with MS. Although most interventions have not been rigorously studied by randomized control trials, they are low-risk, empower the individual by providing self-management techniques, and are affordable. These interventions may be appropriate options for patients with less severe spasticity or may serve as adjunctive treatment for those with more severe spasticity (**Box 2**).

Stretching

Stretching is most often the primary conservative recommendation for spasticity management. An effective active or passive range-of-motion program accomplishes 2 aims: to minimize spasticity-inducing quick stretch of tight muscles, and to preserve range of motion and thus avoid contracture, a secondary complication of spasticity. Although limited data are available on the optimal frequency and type of stretching exercises or splints for spasticity management, weight-bearing stretches appear to be superior to non–weight-bearing stretches, particularly for lower extremity spasticity.[6] In addition, prolonged static stretching appears to have a greater effect.[7] In the patient who cannot perform an adequate active stretching program, range of

Box 1	
Functional measures used in spasticity management	

- Fugl-Meyer
- Arm Activity Measure (ArmA)
- Barthel Index
- Gait speed
- Adductor tone rating scale

Box 2
Conservative modalities for spasticity management

- Stretching: passive, active, static splinting, dynamic splinting, serial casting
- Heat
- Ice
- Vibration
- Electrical stimulation
- Extracorporeal shock-wave therapy

motion may be preserved or improved with serial casting and static or dynamic splinting. Prolonged stretch with casting or splinting may be particularly useful when performed in addition to chemodenervation injections.

Electrical Stimulation

Electrical stimulation has long been recognized for its effects on diminishing spasticity.[8] Stimulation of either antagonists or agonists has been found to produce beneficial effects with reduction of spasticity symptoms. A variety of specific devices have been used for this purpose, including transcutaneous electrical nerve stimulation, functional electrical stimulation, and neuromuscular electrical stimulation. Electrical stimulation also appears to be an effective adjunctive therapy to botulinum toxin injections.[9]

Cryotherapy

For many years, cryotherapy has been known as an effective treatment for spasticity.[10] Cold may be applied in the form of cold baths, cold packs/towels, or vapocoolant sprays. Local application of cryotherapy agents can be applied to agonist or antagonist muscles to treat spasticity. Cold decreases input to the central nervous system by inhibiting sensory afferents; in addition, muscle spindle activity and motor nerve conduction is diminished, resulting in a decrease in spasticity. However, temporary increases in muscle hyperexcitability occur following the application of cryotherapy, which may explain its use in applying treatment to antagonist muscle groups. The effect of icing is short lived, owing to subsequent rewarming of tissues. Cooling may have a general therapeutic effect in patients with MS. In addition, cryotherapy has the benefit of being very accessible and affordable; as Mead and Knott stated eloquently in 1966, "cold is available for the price of ice."[10]

Heat

Although superficial heat (in the form of hot packs, paraffin, diathermy, or infrared application) and deep heat (as applied by ultrasound) have been studied regarding their use in decreasing pain and spasticity in neurologic disorders, there is little objective evidence for the benefit of heat in the literature. The risks of heat therapy in patients with MS must be considered alongside any benefit, given the possibility of heat sensitivity or exacerbation of neurologic symptoms when using heat in this population. In addition, heat must be used with caution in patients with impaired sensation, owing to the risk of burns or injury.

Vibration

Vibration is another well-known modality used to decrease spasticity. Direct application of vibration to a muscle produces contraction of that muscle, and relaxation of the antagonist muscle. This phenomenon is referred to as the tonic vibration reflex.[11] While local muscle vibration has been the mainstay of this therapy, more recently whole-limb and whole-body vibration has been evaluated in small studies, suggesting improvement in spasticity.[12,13]

Extracorporeal Shock-Wave Therapy

A few small studies provide evidence of benefit for shock-wave therapy applied to hypertonic muscles.[14,15] The mechanism of effect of this treatment is unclear, but it has been suggested that extracorporeal shock-wave therapy (ESWT) modifies the characteristics of muscle fibrosis and promotes nitric oxide synthesis.[16] These trials demonstrate significant clinical improvement in spasticity and range of motion following a single treatment of ESWT. The effect of ESWT on spasticity in these studies was found to last for longer than 2 to 3 months. Another recent study compared the additive effect of ESWT with that of electrical stimulation following botulinum toxin injections for spasticity, and found significantly greater improvement in both spasticity and pain in the ESWT group.[17] Of note, ESWT has been evaluated primarily in patients with stroke and cerebral palsy, and not specifically in individuals with MS.

COMPLEMENTARY AND ALTERNATIVE MEDICINE INTERVENTIONS FOR SPASTICITY MANAGEMENT

The use of complementary and alternative medicine (CAM) is highly prevalent in the general population in the United States[18] as well as in individuals with MS. Estimates of prevalence of CAM usage in the MS population range from 54% to 57% in the United States[19,20] and 67.3% in Great Britain.[21] It is important for providers to be familiar with common CAM interventions to facilitate informed discussions with patients. Providers should inquire about adjunctive treatments patients are using, and feel comfortable advising patients on adjunctive treatments or referring patients to reputable sources of information on CAM interventions, such as those available through the National Center for Complementary and Alternative Medicine.

Acupuncture

Among all CAM techniques for spasticity management, acupuncture is likely the most well studied, and demonstrates evidence of benefit for spasticity reduction. Most trials involving acupuncture interventions for spasticity have been performed in the stroke population. Acupuncture has been found to improve spasticity and range of motion in patients with hemiparetic stroke when compared with sham treatments, although significant improvements in quality of life or functional outcome measures were not observed.[22,23] Acupuncture can be performed in isolation, or in combination with adjunctive electrical stimulation or heat with moxibustion.

Cannabis and Cannabinoids

The use of cannabis for spasticity has been recognized and legalized in some states for the treatment of medical conditions, including neurologic disorders, particularly for management of pain and spasticity. Cannabinoids have been found to reduce objective measurements of spasticity in mouse models of MS.[24] Subjective improvement in spasticity and pain symptoms following smoked cannabis has been reported by patients with MS.[25] Similarly, oromucosal delivery of tetrahydrocannabinol extract has shown effectiveness in reducing spasticity symptoms in comparison with placebo.[26]

Other CAM Interventions

Nutritional supplements, massage, chiropractic, and exercise (including yoga) are common forms of CAM used by individuals with MS, but there has been little research on the effect of these treatments specifically on spasticity. A small, uncontrolled clinical trial found no benefit of a yoga intervention on spasticity for patients with MS.[27] Randomized controlled trials investigating the use of fish oil and linoleic acid supplements in patients with MS was assessed in a systematic review, which found no evidence of an effect on global clinical assessments, although spasticity management was not a primary outcome measure. Other interventions, such as reflexology and magnet therapy, have also been described for the control of spasticity, but have limited formal evaluation involving very small clinical trials.[28]

ORAL AND INTRATHECAL MEDICATION MANAGEMENT
Oral Medication

If conservative measures prove inadequate, oral medications can be initiated and are often effective in reducing spasticity. Antispasticity medications can have significant side effects, the most frequently seen being sedation. Therefore, clinicians may opt to trial medications at low doses in the evening to begin with. Baclofen is a good first-line agent that can be initiated in small doses and titrated as needed. Tizanidine is often used as well, as either a first-line or adjunctive agent. The most commonly used medications are discussed here.[2,29–32]

- Baclofen is a γ-aminobutyric acid (GABA)$_B$ agonist that inhibits calcium influx in presynaptic terminals and suppresses release of excitatory neurotransmitters. It inhibits monosynaptic and polysynaptic reflexes, and reduces activity of the γ efferent.
  - Side effects: sedation and slowing of cognition
  - Taper to discontinue: sudden withdrawal can lead to seizures
- Tizanidine is a central α2-agonist that reduces spasticity by increasing presynaptic inhibition of motor neurons.
  - Side effects: sedation, fatigue, slowing of cognition, low blood pressure
  - Monitor liver function
- Benzodiazepines are a class of drugs that facilitate postsynaptic effects of GABA and result in an increase in presynaptic inhibition.
  - Side effects: sedation, fatigue, potential for abuse
  - Taper to discontinue: sudden withdrawal can precipitate seizures
- Dantrolene sodium is the only agent that acts at the muscle level. It reduces release of calcium from the sarcoplasmic reticulum in skeletal muscle (it has little effect on smooth or cardiac muscle).
  - Side effects: muscle weakness, fatigue
  - Monitor liver function

Intrathecal Medication

Baclofen is currently the only antispasticity medication that can be administered intrathecally. It is delivered in liquid form directly into the spinal fluid via an implanted pump system. The literature on intrathecal baclofen (ITB) overwhelmingly supports its effectiveness in reducing spasticity and, in addition, it can be helpful with pain, sleep, and mobility.[33–38] ITB is most effective in managing lower extremity spasticity. The ITB pump has a range of flexible dosing options from a basal-rate adjustment by time of day to bolus infusions.

Before surgical implantation, patients undergo a trial dose of ITB to evaluate how well it will work. The test dose is given via a needle and works in 1 to 2 hours, and wears off in 4 to 8 hours. During this time, evaluation of spasticity, range of motion, and function may be performed to evaluate the efficacy of the drug.[3,33]

The surgical procedure to implant the ITB pump requires general anesthesia and 2 incisions. The first incision is in the lower abdomen, and creates a subcutaneous pocket for the pump. The second incision is in the lower back, and is the insertion site for the catheter to enter the intrathecal space. Typically a flexible silicone catheter is threaded to the level of T10 to T11, but may go as high as T6. The catheter is tunneled under the skin from the back to the lower abdomen, and connected to the pump. The pump needs surgical replacement every 5 to 7 years.[33,39]

The pump itself is a small titanium disk about 3×1 cm in size that has a refillable reservoir for liquid medication, and a computer chip that regulates a battery-operated pump. The pump is refilled transcutaneously every 1 to 3 months on an outpatient basis, and is programmable by a hand-held device. Complications of ITB therapy can include infection, pump or catheter malfunction, and programming error, the latter of which can lead to baclofen overdose or withdrawal.[3,33,39]

CHEMODENERVATION

Peripheral nerve or neuromuscular junction blockade provides an effective and safe means of treating spasticity in MS. Peripheral injections have the advantage of eliminating the side effects of oral spasticity medications. In addition, the duration of effect for peripheral injections is relatively long. Injections are ideal for addressing focal rather than generalized spasticity symptoms, such as hip adductor spasticity.

As an invasive procedure, however, spasticity injections are not without risk, and require operator skill to maximize benefit and minimize associated risks. In particular, chemical neurolysis with phenol requires practitioner expertise for nerve or motor endplate localization. Treatment plans may be affected by considerations of cost and maximum total dose per session. Patient factors to consider include compliance with a home exercise program, patient preference, diagnosis, duration of disease, and prognosis.

Any injection requires the practitioner's decision on the choice of neurolytic agent and choice of muscles to inject. Botulinum toxin is the most commonly used agent for chemodenervation; however, phenol is also used and has some advantages over botulinum toxin in particular cases. Phenol is much less expensive than botulinum toxin, has an immediate onset of action and longer duration of effect, can be repeated frequently if needed, and can be effective for managing spasticity in large muscle groups. The disadvantages of phenol neurolysis are increased time required for peripheral nerve or motor point identification during the procedure, the potential for painful dysthesthesias when injecting mixed motor and sensory nerves, and increased complexity with subsequent injections arising from scarring and muscle fibrosis.

Once the desired neurolytic agent is determined, target muscles for injection may be identified through the patient's primary functional complaints, goals of treatment, and examination findings suggesting culprit muscles. A treatment plan should be drafted before initiation of the injection procedure, with the targeted muscles and doses designated for the procedure.

Occasionally patients present with such severe spasticity that it is difficult to tease apart the spastic component of the range-of-motion limitations from the soft-tissue contracture. This critical distinction can have a great impact on further treatment decisions. In this scenario, a diagnostic nerve block with anesthetic agent, performed with localization using a peripheral nerve stimulator, can subdue the spastic component and permit examination to determine limitations resulting from soft-tissue contracture. Should an adequate peripheral nerve blockade reveal no change in range-of-motion limitation, this would suggest that the major component of the limitation is due to soft-tissue contracture rather than spasticity, and chemodenervation would likely be of limited benefit. However, if peripheral nerve blockade reveals great improvement in the range of motion, this would indicate that the target muscles supplied by this nerve may be amenable to chemodenervation, thus to improve the range of motion in that region. Peripheral nerve blockade may also be useful to identify culprit muscles producing the most limiting spasticity in regions where multiple nerve territories overlap individual joints, such as the hand.

In addition to anatomic localization, several tools are available for the practitioner to maximize accuracy and confirm the intended localization of the injection. Such tools include electromyography, peripheral nerve stimulation, and ultrasonography. Electromyography is the most commonly used tool for localization, likely because of its widespread availability and training among physiatrists. Use of electromyography confirms intramuscular delivery of the injectate, but cannot distinguish individual muscles in the patient that cannot selectively activate the targeted muscle. Peripheral nerve stimulation is helpful in selectively identifying smaller muscles when the patient is unable to initiate movement, or when precise localization of the nerve or motor endplate is desired; this is particularly useful for phenol or alcohol neurolysis. Ultrasonography provides real-time visualization of the anatomy, with the additional benefit of identifying adjacent structures such as neurovascular bundles, which can be useful in avoiding complication. Adjunctive treatment is paramount to the success of spasticity interventions via injection. Several studies have evaluated the efficacy of adding treatment with neuromuscular electrical stimulation, functional electrical stimulation, stretching, dynamic splinting, serial casting, constraint-induced movement therapy, or body-weight–supported treadmill training to botulinum toxin treatment, with additional benefit being shown.[40]

CASE STUDY EXAMPLES

For Patient A, the woman in our first case, examination and history showed a focal spasticity. Strength in the right leg was 5/5 except for dorsiflexion, which was 4/5, and her gastrocnemius muscle was noted to have tone of MAS 1+. Her gait was significant for right toe scuffing and slight circumduction of right leg. Initial treatment included an aggressive stretching regimen and functional electrical stimulator ankle foot orthosis. As the years progressed, she required more intervention in the form of botulinum toxin to the gastrocnemius muscle. She never required oral medication.

For Patient B, the man in our second case, examination and history showed more diffuse bilateral lower extremity spasticity. He had 1/5 to 2/5 muscle strength, MAS 2 in quadriceps, and MAS 3 in adductors. Workup for any precipitating factors, including constipation, urinary retention, urinary tract infection, renal or bladder calculi, infection, skin ulcers, or other acute medical conditions, was negative. Treatment included modifying his environment to have comfortable temperature, no restrictive clothing, and a specialty mattress with head and leg adjustments. His daily care plan increased to aggressive stretching twice a day. He trialed many conservative treatments, including bracing, electrical stimulation, and acupuncture. He was unable to tolerate additional oral medication because of significant side effects. He underwent chemodenervation of bilateral adductors without success. Ultimately his spasticity was managed by a combination of conservative measures and an ITB pump with a variable basal dosing regimen to accommodate higher concentrations at night.

SUMMARY

Spasticity can manifest in many different ways clinically, and can have multiple triggers. Evaluation involves taking a thorough history, performing a physical examination, and rating functional impairment. Management starts with treating any underlying medical conditions, modifying any precipitating triggers, forming a daily care plan of stretching and exercise, and making use of physical modalities and CAM. If needed, more aggressive management can include oral medication, chemodenervation, intrathecal medication, and surgical interventions.

REFERENCES

1. Rizzo MA, Hadjimichael OC, Preiningerova J, et al. Prevalence and treatment of spasticity reported by multiple sclerosis patients. Mult Scler 2004;10:589–95.
2. Samkoff LM, Goodman AD. Symptomatic management in multiple sclerosis. Neurol Clin 2011;29(2):449–63.
3. Kheder A, Nair KP. Spasticity: pathophysiology, evaluation and management. Pract Neurol 2012;12(5):289–98.
4. Lance JW. 1980 symposium synopsis. In: Feldman RG, Young RR, Koella WP, editors. Spasticity: disordered motor control. Chicago: Year Book Medical Publishers; 1980. p. 485–94.
5. Sheean G, McGuire JR. Spastic hypertonia and movement disorders: pathophysiology, clinical presentation, and quantification. PM R 2009;1:827–33.
6. Odéen I, Knutsson E. Evaluation of the effects of muscle stretch and weight load in patients with spastic paraplegia. Scand J Rehabil Med 1981;13:117–21.
7. Odéen I. Reduction of muscular hypertonus by long-term muscle stretch. Scand J Rehabil Med 1981;13:93–9.
8. Levine MG, Knott M, Kabat H. Relaxation of spasticity by electrical stimulation of antagonist muscles. Arch Phys Med Rehabil 1952;33:668–73.
9. Hesse S, Reiter F, Konrad M, et al. Botulinum toxin type A and short-term electrical stimulation in the treatment of upper limb flexor spasticity after stroke: a randomized, double-blind, placebo-controlled trial. Clin Rehabil 1998;12:381–8.
10. Mead S, Knott M. Topical cryotherapy: use for relief of pain and spasticity. Calif Med 1966;105:179–81.
11. Eklund G, Hagbarth KE. Motor effects of vibratory muscle stimuli in man. Electroencephalogr Clin Neurophysiol 1965;19:619.
12. Ahlborg L, Andersson C, Julin P. Whole-body vibration training compared with resistance training: effect on spasticity, muscle strength and motor performance in adults with cerebral palsy. J Rehabil Med 2006;38:302–8.
13. Ness L, Field-Fote E. Effect of whole-body vibration on quadriceps spasticity in individuals with spastic hypertonia due to spinal cord injury. Restor Neurol Neurosci 2009;27:623–33.
14. Manganotti P, Amelio E. Long-term effect of shock wave therapy on upper limb hypertonia in patients affected by stroke. Stroke 2005;36:1967–71.
15. Vidal X, Morral A, Costa L, et al. Radial extracorporeal shock wave therapy (rESWT) in the treatment of spasticity in cerebral palsy: a randomized, placebo-controlled clinical trial. NeuroRehabilitation 2011;29:413–9.

16. Mariotto S, Cavalieri E, Amelio E, et al. Extracorporeal shock waves: from lithotripsy to anti-inflammatory action by NO production. Nitric Oxide 2005;12: 89–96.

17. Santamato A, Notarnicola A, Panza F, et al. SBOTE study: extracorporeal shock wave therapy versus electrical stimulation after botulinum toxin type A injection for post-stroke spasticity—a prospective randomized trial. Ultrasound Med Biol 2013;39:283–91.

18. Eisenberg D, Davis R, Ettner S, et al. Trends in alternative medicine use in the United States, 1990-1997: results of a follow-up national survey. JAMA 1998; 280:1569–75.

19. Marrie RA, Hadjimichael O, Vollmer T. Predictors of alternative medicine use by multiple sclerosis patients. Mult Scler 2003;9:461–6.

20. Nayak S, Matheis RJ, Schoenberger NE. Use of unconventional therapies by individuals with multiple sclerosis. Clin Rehabil 2003;17:181–91.

21. Apel A, Greim B, König N, et al. Frequency of current utilisation of complementary and alternative medicine by patients with multiple sclerosis. J Neurol 2006;253: 1331–6.

22. Mukherjee M, McPeak LK, Redford JB, et al. The effect of electro-acupuncture on spasticity of the wrist joint in chronic stroke survivors. Arch Phys Med Rehabil 2007;88:159–66.

23. Wayne PM, Krebs DE, Mackin EA. Acupuncture for upper-extremity rehabilitation in chronic stroke: a randomized Sham-controlled study. Arch Phys Med Rehabil 2005;86:2248–55.

24. Arévalo-Martín Á, Vela JM, Molina Holgado E, et al. Therapeutic action of cannabinoids in a murine model of multiple sclerosis. J Neurosci 2003;23:2511–6.

25. Consroe P, Musty R, Rein J, et al. The perceived effects of smoked cannabis on patients with multiple sclerosis. Eur Neurol 1997;38:44–8.

26. Wade DT, Makela P, Robson P. Do cannabis-based medicinal extracts have general or specific effects on symptoms in multiple sclerosis? A double-blind, randomized, placebo-controlled study on 160 patients. Mult Scler 2004;10: 434–41.

27. Velikonja O, Čurić K, Ožura A, et al. Influence of sports climbing and yoga on spasticity, cognitive function, mood and fatigue in patients with multiple sclerosis. Clin Neurol Neurosurg 2002;112:597–601.

28. Huntley A, Ernst E. Complementary and alternative therapies for treating multiple sclerosis symptoms: a systematic review. Complement Ther Med 2002;8:97–105.

29. Multiple Sclerosis Council for Clinical Practice Guidelines. Spasticity management in multiple sclerosis: evidence-based management strategies for spasticity. Treatment in multiple sclerosis: clinical practice guidelines 2003. J Spinal Cord Med 2005;28:167–99.

30. Markowitz C. Symptomatic therapy of multiple sclerosis. CONTINUUM: lifelong learning in neurology. Continuum (Minneap Minn) 2010;16(5 Multiple Sclerosis): 90–104.

31. Watanabe T. Spasticity: role of oral medications in spasticity management. PM R 2009;1:839–41.

32. Malanga G, Reiter RD, Garay E. Update on tizanidine for muscle spasticity and emerging indications. Expert Opin Pharmacother 2008;9:2209–15.

33. Francisco GE, Saulino MF, Yablon SA, et al. Intrathecal baclofen therapy: an update. PM R 2009;1:852–8.

34. Rekand T, Gronning M. Treatment of spasticity related to multiple sclerosis with intrathecal baclofen: a long-term follow-up. J Rehabil Med 2011;43:511–4.

35. Saval A, Chiodo A. Intrathecal baclofen for spasticity management: a comparative analysis of spasticity of spinal vs cortical origin. J Spinal Cord Med 2010; 33:16–21.

36. Dario A, Tomei G. Management of spasticity in multiple sclerosis by intrathecal baclofen. Acta Neurochir Suppl 2007;97:189–92.

37. Vender JR, Hughes M, Hughes BD, et al. Intrathecal baclofen therapy and multiple sclerosis: outcomes and patient satisfaction. Neurosurg Focus 2006;21:1–4.

38. Bensmail D, Quera Salva MA, Roche N, et al. Effect of intrathecal baclofen on sleep and respiratory function in patients with spasticity. Neurology 2006;67: 1432–6.

39. Medtronic. Synchromed II: programmable infusion system clinical reference guide. Available at: http://professional.medtronic.com/wcm/groups/mdtcom_sg/@mdt/@neuro/documents/documents/itb-surg-proc.pdf. Accessed January 15, 2013.

40. Elovic EP, Esquenazi A, Alter K, et al. Chemodenervation and nerve blocks in the diagnosis and management of spasticity and muscle overactivity. PM R 2009;1: 842–51.

Exercise in Multiple Sclerosis

Alexius E.G. Sandoval, MD

KEYWORDS

- Multiple • Sclerosis • Exercise • Resistance • Endurance • Training

KEY POINTS

- Exercise is an intervention that may be used in the management of multiple sclerosis (MS).
- Certain exercise physiology characteristics are commonly seen among persons with MS, particularly in the more debilitated.
- Studies have shown numerous beneficial effects of exercise in MS.
- There are general guidelines that may be followed for proper exercise prescription for the MS population.
- There are several recommendations that may help improve the quality of future MS exercise trials.

INTRODUCTION

Views regarding exercise in persons with MS have been evolving over the years. The old paradigm was to discourage persons with MS from exercising to avoid increases in core body temperature that would exacerbate MS-related signs and symptoms.[1–3] It was believed that this strategy would conserve energy and make it available for activities of daily living (ADLs).[3] Furthermore, because fatigue is a common symptom in MS, it was previously thought that fatigue would prevent persons with MS from tolerating much exercise.[1] The more recent paradigm is to encourage an appropriate level of exercise in persons with MS in an effort to reduce MS-related symptoms and to promote general wellness.

The impairments seen in MS may result from either the disease process per se or from deconditioning.[3–8] Impairments from the disease process itself (ie, due to demyelination and axonal degeneration) are probably not reversible with exercise. Impairments from deconditioning (ie, as a consequence of reduced physical activity levels) are probably reversible with exercise.

There are well-known detrimental effects of a general lack of exercise. A sedentary lifestyle is strongly associated with increased morbidity and mortality rates among

Department of Rehabilitation Medicine, Eastern Maine Medical Center, 905 Union Street, Suite 9, Bangor, ME 04401, USA
E-mail address: aesandoval@emh.org

Phys Med Rehabil Clin N Am 24 (2013) 605–618
http://dx.doi.org/10.1016/j.pmr.2013.06.010
1047-9651/13/$ – see front matter © 2013 Elsevier Inc. All rights reserved.

pmr.theclinics.com

non-MS adults.[9–11] These individuals have an increased risk of developing chronic health problems, such as obesity, cardiovascular disease,[1] type 2 diabetes, cancer, osteoporosis, and fatigue.[3,12,13] Physiologically, these individuals have reduced aerobic capacity, decreased muscle strength, and increased muscle atrophy.[3,14,15]

Similar findings are seen among persons with MS, with the more sedentary individuals displaying an increased incidence of cardiovascular disease, osteoporosis, and obesity.[9,16–21] Other preexisting MS-related symptoms, such as depression and fatigue, may worsen.[1,3] Very low activity levels in persons with MS often coincide with a loss in leisure activities, social contacts, or usual ADLs that are important for self-esteem and psychological well-being.[1,5,6]

Conversely, there are well-documented benefits of increased physical activity and exercise. Physical activity is associated with the following benefits: decreased risk of chronic health problems (such as cardiovascular disease, diabetes, osteoporosis, obesity, and depression), decreased incidence of premature mortality, and favorable effects on mental health.[9,22–24]

Given the overwhelming recommendations promoting increased physical activity and exercise in the general population, there has been great interest to determine if similar recommendations may be applied to persons with MS and reap similar benefits.

PHYSIOLOGIC CHARACTERISTICS OF PERSONS WITH MS

Studies have searched for characteristics unique among persons with MS in terms of cardiovascular and muscle physiology that are distinct from those of the general population. It may be difficult to generalize these characteristics among all persons with MS given the wide spectrum of prevalent impairments and disabilities. Specific MS-related physiologic characteristics likely are most evident in the more severely debilitated, whereas those with only mild MS may not be too physiologically different from their healthy, age-matched counterparts.

Generally speaking, and again these may be more evident in more debilitated individuals, the following physiologic characteristics were noted among persons with MS:

1. Decreased aerobic capacity (maximum oxygen consumption [$\dot{V}O_2max$]),[3,25,26] which was approximately 30% lower than in healthy controls[27]; even greater deficits were seen in maximum work rate at aerobic threshold, which suggests a very low training level and marked deconditioning[26,27]
2. Decreased maximal muscle strength, both during isokinetic[3,28–31] and isometric[3,7,8,28,32–38] muscle contractions, with strength impairment more prominent in the lower extremities than in the upper extremities[3,36]
3. Reduced comfortable and maximal gait velocity[3,39,40]
4. Lower health-related quality of life (HRQL)[3,41]

The following physiologic characteristics of persons with MS were inconsistent among various studies and are harder to generalize:

1. Increased resting heart rate[3,25,42–44]
2. Increased diastolic blood pressure[3,42,44]
3. Increased muscle atrophy[3,7,8,31]
4. Decreased rate of force development[3,32–35,38]
5. Decreased muscle mass[3,7,8,31,32,45,46]
6. Decreased fat-free mass at the whole-body level[3,45,46]
7. Shifts in muscle fiber–type composition from type I to type IIa and IIax (as seen in immobilized non-MS individuals)[3,46,47]

EXERCISE PHYSIOLOGY AND MS
Aerobic Capacity

Maximal aerobic capacity is influenced by the degree of physical impairment in persons with MS. Those with greater impairments can only exercise for a shorter period and can only achieve a lower maximal exercise intensity and lower $\dot{V}o_2$max. Aerobic capacity is limited by respiratory muscle dysfunction and deconditioning.[27,48–50]

Among persons with MS who are paraplegic, the upper limbs impose an upper limit to aerobic performance.[27,51,52] Thus, these individuals with limited lower extremity function due to weakness, spasticity, or cerebellar dysfunction may not be able to increase their metabolic rate enough to improve aerobic fitness. Their residual functional muscle mass may be too small to take up enough oxygen to get a cardiovascular workout.[27,53] Thus, the goal of aerobic exercise for the severely impaired should be more maintenance rather than improvement of cardiovascular fitness.[27]

Cardiovascular Dysautonomia

More debilitated persons with MS may exhibit cardiovascular dysautonomia. This is seen as a blunted heart rate and blood pressure response to exercise.[54,55] Regarding blunted blood pressure response, there may be an attenuated rise in blood pressure during exercise.[44,54,56] This may lead to insufficient perfusion of brain or muscle and premature development of exertional symptoms, such as lightheadedness or muscle fatigue. Thus heart rate, blood pressure, and clinical symptoms should be carefully monitored in MS individuals with known or suspected cardiovascular dysautonomia.

Muscle Strength and Endurance

Persons with MS typically have less muscle strength compared with healthy controls,[28,29,35,54–60] a slower rate of muscle tension, and reduced muscle endurance.[36,54] In mild cases of MS, however, muscle function is close to normal.[27]

Flexibility

Persons with MS often have decreased flexibility, especially in those with spasticity. This has to be properly assessed and taken into consideration when designing the exercise prescription.[54]

Heat Intolerance

A frequent concern with exercise in MS is potentially triggering Uhthoff phenomenon. Uhthoff phenomenon was originally described as a transient amblyopia due to overheating from exercise.[27,61] The term has since been expanded to include other symptoms triggered by overheating.[27,62] The exact mechanism of Uhthoff phenomenon is unclear. It may be due to heat-worsened conduction across partially demyelinated axons, fatigue of damaged neuronal pathways with repetitive nerve transmission,[27,63] or a hormonal factor produced with cooling.[4,64]

Exercise-induced Uhthoff phenomenon should not be regarded as a contraindication to exercise.[27] It is usually reversible and often resolves within an hour or even sooner with rapid cooling.[27] Furthermore, it is still more common for heating to produce just general fatigue than an Uhthoff phenomenon with focal neurologic deficits.[27,49]

How much does the body temperature change with exercise? Studies have shown that routine exercise does not significantly increase core body temperature.

Ponichtera-Mulcare and colleagues[55] noted a mean rectal temperature change of 0.1°C during land-based exercise and −0.1°C during water-based exercise.[27] Alternatively, normal thermoregulatory reflexes (eg, sweating and vasodilatation) that maintain a steady core temperature during routine exercise may be impaired in persons with MS. In such cases, a rise in core temperature of even less than 1°C may be enough to trigger heat-related symptoms.[27,65]

The use of cooling devices and strategies seems to provide some modest benefits for persons with MS. One such device, used by Capello and colleagues[66] and Kraft and Alquist,[67] was a head-vest liquid cooling garment. The former found a slight improvement in pyramidal and cerebellar function[27] whereas the latter demonstrated a treatment effect for strength, dynamic coordination, and endurance capacity, with greater heat loss associated with greater motor function gain.[27,67] Syndulko and colleagues[68] saw reduced fatigue and improved ambulation for up to 3 hours postcooling with the use of either the liquid cooling system or an icepack suit.[27]

When engaging in pool-based exercises, the ideal pool temperature for heat-sensitive MS individuals seems between 27°C and 29°C (80°F–84°F).[27,54,69] Temperatures below 27°C can paradoxically increase spasticity.[27,70]

BENEFITS OF EXERCISE IN MS

The general consensus from research to date is that there are many benefits associated with regular physical activity and/or exercise training in persons with MS.[1,9,57,71,72] These benefits are comparable to those seen in healthy, non-MS individuals.

A Cochrane review evaluated the evidence for exercise therapy for MS.[1] Of all published studies on the topic at the time, the review found only 9 high-quality randomized controlled trials. Analysis of these 9 randomized controlled trials yielded the following conclusions:

1. There was strong evidence for a beneficial effect of exercise on muscle power functions (isometric strength), exercise tolerance functions (physical fitness), and mobility-related activities.
2. There was moderate evidence for a beneficial effect of exercise on upper extremity function and mood.
3. There was no evidence for a beneficial effect of exercise on the Expanded Disability Status Scale (EDSS), fatigue, cognitive impairment, ADLs/instrumental ADLs, HRQL, blood lipids, and body composition.

This Cochrane review also determined that no 1 MS exercise program was any more successful than other (control) exercises,[1] regarding the outcome measures of physical fitness, mobility, fatigue, and HRQL. There was little evidence to support any particular exercise program as superior for persons with MS.[9]

These study findings, however, may not be readily generalizable to more severely disabled MS individuals. The majority of exercise trials only recruited MS subjects with low to moderate disabilities (EDSS<7).[9,27] More disabled MS individuals may not benefit as much from exercise because (1) they may not be able to activate enough muscle mass to generate a training effect, (2) the exercise programs may not be properly designed for them, and (3) their adherence may be poor.[27] For these individuals, a better strategy may be a multidisciplinary outpatient program rather than exercise alone.[27] Such a strategy should be focused more on function maintenance rather than improvement.

EXERCISE TRAINING: RESISTANCE, ENDURANCE, AND COMBINED TRAINING

There are 2 major types of exercises studied in MS exercise trials. These are resistance and endurance exercises. There are also a few studies that investigated the effects of a combination of both resistance and endurance exercises.

Resistance Exercises

Resistance exercises use few muscle contractions against a heavy load with the goal of increasing muscle strength.[3] There are several studies on the effects of resistance training on muscle strength and function in MS.[54] There are, however, fewer studies on resistance training compared with endurance training in the MS population.[3] The few resistance exercise studies in MS are often of low methodological quality, used only moderate training intensities with mild progression, and only included subjects with mild to moderate MS (EDSS<6.5). Although these studies were of heterogeneous designs, the general conclusion is that resistance training of moderate intensity produced improvements in muscle strength and some functional measures among moderately impaired persons with MS.[3,73–80] Resistance exercises were generally safe and well tolerated.[3]

Endurance Exercises

Endurance exercises use multiple muscle contractions against a low load with the goal of increasing aerobic capacity.[3] Endurance training is more extensively studied in the MS population than resistance training.[3] The training regimens used in these studies were often insufficiently described, the training intensities used were poorly controlled (but usually described as low to moderate), and the subjects only had mild to moderate MS (EDSS<7).[3] The training modalities used were heterogeneous, including bicycle ergometry, arm ergometry, arm-leg ergometry, aquatic exercise, and treadmill walking. In general, endurance training of low to moderate intensity produced improvements in aerobic capacity and in measures of HRQL, mood, and depression in persons with mild to moderate MS (EDSS<7).[3] Endurance training was generally safe and well tolerated.[3]

Endurance training produces significant adaptations of the cardiorespiratory and neuromuscular systems that enhance the delivery of oxygen from the atmosphere to the mitochondria and enable a tighter regulation of muscle metabolism.[3,81] Individuals with MS have been shown to make favorable gains in cardiorespiratory fitness within a short span of 4 weeks.[26,54]

Combined Resistance and Endurance Exercises

There are few studies investigating the effects of combined resistance and endurance training in the MS population. Dalgas and colleagues[3] found in their review only 2 qualified randomized controlled trials. Combined training produced small improvements in muscle strength and functional capacity (gait velocity). No changes were seen, however, in aerobic capacity, depression, fatigue, and HRQL.[82–85] Combined training was generally safe and well tolerated.[3]

EXERCISE PRESCRIPTION GUIDELINES

Several published articles offer general guidelines on exercise prescription for the MS population. These guidelines are summarized as follows.

Exercise Staircase Model

Brown and Kraft proposed an exercise staircase model for exercise prescription and progression for a broad spectrum of MS individuals.[27]

At the bottom of the staircase is passive range-of-motion exercises. This serves as the foundation and is appropriate for the most physically and cognitively disabled. These exercises should be performed at least once a day.

The next step up the staircase is active range-of-motion exercises. These are appropriate for less disabled MS individuals and may be performed with or without gravity eliminated as strength allows. Even when weakness is diffuse, resistance exercises of carefully selected muscles, probably not more than 2 per limb, may still allow effective strengthening. In motivated individuals with mild MS, focused muscle strengthening with progressive resistive exercises may be effective.

The third and highest step in the staircase is integrated exercises. Integrated exercises use a combination of strength, endurance, balance, coordination, and flexibility exercises. The exact combination of exercises is tailored to individual needs and capabilities. Aquatic exercise is a good example of an integrated exercise.

Pre-exercise Screening

A thorough pre-exercise evaluation should be performed before designing an individualized exercise program. Ideally this is done by an expert in the field who has experience working with MS individuals. This may be a physical therapist, exercise physiologist,[3,9,27,54] or physical medicine and rehabilitation physician. Attention should be given to an individual's chief complaint and reason for exercise referral, which may be fatigue, weakness, imbalance, incoordination, and so forth.[9] The evaluation should include a thorough physical examination and history, including MS, functional, and exercise histories.

A cardiopulmonary function review should also be done.[1,62] Some investigators have recommended getting a baseline EKG or submaximal stress test.[86] There are others who do not find getting such tests always necessary unless indicated by individual cardiovascular risk factors and cardiac history.[27] The individual's other existing medical comorbidities should also be taken into consideration, such as cardiovascular disease, musculoskeletal or mental disorders, obesity, and the exercise program modified accordingly.[9,20,21,87,88]

Petajan and White further classify MS individuals into the following functional categories: (1) normal (no fatigue or heat sensitivity), (2) normal with fatigue, (3) mild to moderate motor disability, and (4) severe motor disability.[9,62] Such classification may further help tailor the exercise prescription.

Exercise Prescription

The individualized exercise prescription is designed to address a patient's chief complaint or goal—to improve strength, endurance, balance, coordination, fatigue, and so forth. It should take into account a patient's baseline impairments and capabilities.[9,54] The prescription should include all the necessary components, such as frequency, duration, intensity, modalities to be used, and precautions to be observed.[9] Examples of common precautions in MS include fall risk, motor fatigue necessitating rest breaks, heat sensitivity, and cognitive changes that may limit learning or safety awareness. Because MS-related symptoms and impairments may fluctuate or worsen over time, the MS individual has to be periodically reassessed and the exercise program modified accordingly.

Pre-exercise Cool Down

Particularly for individuals with heat sensitivity, several investigators have recommended pre-exercise cooling strategies, such as the use of cooling devices,[2,9,62,89] cold water lower body immersion,[2,54] or taking a tepid bath 20 to 30 minutes before (and after) exercise.[27] Individuals should wear light exercise clothing or may even try exercising with a cooling vest. The exercise area temperature should be kept cool through the use of fans or air conditioning.[27]

Flexibility and Stretching

Individuals with MS often have decreased joint range of motion due to spasticity and prolonged immobility. The goals of flexibility exercises are to increase muscle length, increase joint mobility, counteract the effects of spasticity, and improve posture and balance.[54] Flexibility exercises should be performed at least daily for 10 to 15 minutes.[54,90] Stretching should be done before and after workout sessions and should include the upper and lower body muscle groups used in the workout. Spastic muscles should be particularly targeted.

Stretches should be slow, gentle, and prolonged. There should be no bouncing with the stretch. The stretch should be up to the end of the comfort range and held there for 20 to 60 seconds. Stretching should not be painful. Individuals who need help with stretching may use a towel, rope, or partner. For immobilized individuals with spasticity, passive stretching may be done by a therapist or trained caregiver. For higher-functioning MS individuals, stretching exercises may be done through a supervised yoga class.[54,91,92]

Exercise Intensity

Brown and Kraft[27] recommended exercising below maximal workload as a reasonable safeguard to avoid undue cardiac stress, fatigue, and Uhthoff phenomenon. To achieve an exercise intensity of approximately 55% to 60% $\dot{V}o_2max$, the target heart rate for most MS individuals may be computed as $(220 - age) \times (0.7)$. For MS individuals with marked deconditioning or heat sensitivity, the target heart rate may be computed as $(220 - age) \times (0.65)$.

These formulae may not be applicable to the more severely disabled MS individuals with cardiovascular dysautonomia and blunted heart rate responses. For these individuals, the target exercise intensity may be better estimated by aiming for a Borg Rating of Perceived Exertion level of 11 to 14, or moderate intensity.[9,54] Morrison and colleagues[93] found that the (modified) Borg Rating of Perceived Exertion scale and other physiologic responses to submaximal and maximal exercise were similar between MS participants and healthy controls.[9] This is despite MS participants reporting higher levels of fatigue than controls.

Resistance Training

It is recommended that resistance training be performed under the supervision of experienced personnel for safety until the MS individual is comfortable with the training program.[3] Additionally, it has been shown that supervised is superior to nonsupervised resistance training.[3,94]

In terms of resistance training modalities, it is recommended that an individual start off using training machines (ie, closed kinetic chains) instead of free weights (ie, open kinetic chains) for safety.[3] If training machines are unavailable, alternatives include the use of elastic bands and body weight as load.

Training frequency should be 2 to 3 days per week. Training intensity should be in the range of 8 to 15 repetition maximum (RM), with initial starting intensities approximately 15 RM. This should gradually be increased over several months toward intensities of approximately 8 to 10 RM. Resistance can be safely increased by 2% to 5% when 15 repetitions are correctly performed in consecutive training sessions.[54,75] The rate of progression should allow for full recovery between training sessions to prevent musculoskeletal overuse injuries.[54] The individual should start with 1 to 3 sets, which can be gradually increased over a few months to 3 to 4 sets of each exercise. Allow rest breaks of 2 to 4 minutes between sets and exercises.

In terms of number of exercises, a whole-body program containing 4 to 8 exercises is recommended. In general, exercise large muscle groups before small muscle groups, and perform multiple-joint exercises before single-joint exercises.[3,95] Prioritize lower extremity over upper extremity exercises. It has been shown that in MS individuals the lower extremity strength deficit is greater than that of the upper extremity.[3,36] Make sure to include legs, back, shoulders, chest, and arms, observing any contraindications based on individual impairments.[54]

In terms of precautions, weight lifting should be done in a seated position (as in most weight machines) to minimize the risk of falls with free weights. If an individual has impaired proprioception or coordination, the exercise should be done under supervision.[54]

Endurance Training

Recommended endurance training modalities include bicycle ergometry, arm-leg ergometry, arm ergometry, treadmill walking, and aquatic exercise.[3,54] For higher-functioning MS individuals, additional options include the treadmill, elliptical, running, and rowing.

Training frequency should be 2 to 3 times per week. Training duration should be 10 to 40 minutes, depending on the level of disability. Training intensity should initially begin with approximately 50% to 70% $\dot{V}o_2$max, corresponding to 60% to 80% of maximum heart rate. If an individual has a blunted heart rate response, an alternative measure is to aim for a Borg Rating of Perceived Exertion level of 11 to 14, or moderate intensity.[54]

In terms of training progression, previously sedentary individuals should start aerobic exercises at a comfortable level and then increase the intensity and duration at weekly or monthly intervals.[27,96] For the first 2 to 6 months, the training volume may be increased by either prolonging the training duration or by adding an extra training day. After this period, it should be tested whether the individual can tolerate a higher training intensity. This can be done by replacing 1 training session with interval training using intensities of up to 90% $\dot{V}o_2$max.

Combined Resistance and Endurance Training

Resistance training may need to be done first before endurance training, particularly among MS individuals with significant strength deficits.[3,54] Muscle strength deficits may limit the ability of MS individuals to engage in aerobic exercise of sufficient intensity and duration to enhance cardiorespiratory fitness.[54] Thus, initial resistance training may make subsequent endurance training possible for such individuals.

Training frequency should be 2 days per week of resistance training alternating with 2 days per week of endurance training. These exercise periods should be separated by an interval of 24 to 48 hours to allow for recovery.[5,90]

RECOMMENDATIONS FOR FUTURE RESEARCH

There are several common recommendations for future research proposed by currently available studies. These include the following.

1. Subjects: Stratify subjects on the basis of MS types and degree of disability (EDSS). Studies should recruit subjects with greater disability (EDSS>6.5), including

semiambulatory and nonambulatory individuals, those with longer durations of MS, and more elderly MS individuals.

2. Methodology: Ideally there should be larger sample sizes, proper blinding, randomization, and accounting for all dropouts. Longer exercise training periods (>12 weeks) should be used to adequately detect a training effect.[3,97]

3. Interventions: More studies on resistance training and combined resistance and endurance training programs are needed.[3] More detailed descriptions of the training regimen used should be provided in published articles to allow for better reproducibility and comparison among studies.[3] Different training intensities should be evaluated to see if MS individuals could tolerate and benefit from more intense training.[3]

4. Measures: Reach a consensus on a core set of standardized outcome measures to be used in exercise trials.[1] At present, individual exercise trials use varying outcome measures, making result comparison and generalization difficult. Ideally, outcome measures should routinely include measures of ADLs and HRQL.

SUMMARY

Exercise offers many benefits for persons with MS, just as it does for the general population. Certain exercise physiology characteristics are commonly seen among persons with MS, particularly in the more debilitated. Properly prescribed exercise programs can improve modifiable impairments in MS. Exercise is generally safe and well tolerated. There are general guidelines that may be followed for exercise prescription for the MS population. The quality of MS exercise trials may be improved by applying several recommendations.

REFERENCES

1. Rietberg MB, Brooks D, Uitdehaag BM, et al. Exercise therapy for multiple sclerosis. Cochrane Database Syst Rev 2004;(3):CD003980.
2. White AT, Wilson TE, Davis SL, et al. Effect of precooling on physical performance in multiple sclerosis. Mult Scler 2000;6(3):176–80.
3. Dalgas U, Stenager E, Ingemann-Hansen T. Multiple sclerosis and physical exercise: recommendations for the application of resistance-, endurance-, and combined training. Mult Scler 2008;14(1):35–53.
4. de Ruiter CJ, Jongen PJ, van der Woude LH, et al. Contractile speed and fatigue of adductor pollicis muscle in multiple sclerosis. Muscle Nerve 2001; 24(9):1173–80.
5. Ng AV, Kent-Braun JA. Quantitation of lower physical activity in persons with multiple sclerosis. Med Sci Sports Exerc 1997;29(4):517–23.
6. Stuifbergen AK. Physical activity and perceived health status in persons with multiple sclerosis. J Neurosci Nurs 1997;29(4):238–43.
7. Garner DJ, Widrick JJ. Cross-bridge mechanisms of muscle weakness in multiple sclerosis. Muscle Nerve 2003;27(4):456–64.
8. Kent-Braun JA, Ng AV, Castro M, et al. Strength, skeletal muscle composition, and enzyme activity in multiple sclerosis. J Appl Physiol 1997;83(6):1998–2004.
9. Vollmer T, Benedict R, Bennett S, et al. Exercise as prescriptive therapy in multiple sclerosis: a consensus conference white paper. Int J MS Care 2012; 14(Suppl 3):2–14.
10. Garber AJ. Obesity and type 2 diabetes: which patients are at risk? Diabetes Obes Metab 2012;14(5):399–408.

11. Thorp AA, Owen N, Neuhaus M, et al. Sedentary behaviors and subsequent health outcomes in adults: a systematic review of longitudinal studies, 1996-2011. Am J Prev Med 2011;41(2):207–15.
12. Pedersen BK, Saltin B. Evidence for prescribing exercise as therapy in chronic disease. Scand J Med Sci Sports 2006;16(Suppl 1):3–63.
13. Berlin AA, Kop WJ, Deuster PA. Depressive mood symptoms and fatigue after exercise withdrawal: the potential role of decreased fitness. Psychosom Med 2006;68(2):224–30.
14. Convertino VA. Cardiovascular consequences of bed rest: effect on maximal oxygen uptake. Med Sci Sports Exerc 1997;29(2):191–6.
15. Convertino VA, Bloomfield SA, Greenleaf JE. An overview of the issues: physiological effects of bed rest and restricted physical activity. Med Sci Sports Exerc 1997;29(2):187–90.
16. Motl R, Goldman M. Physical inactivity, neurological disability, and cardiorespiratory fitness in multiple sclerosis. Acta Neurol Scand 2011;123(2):98–104.
17. Ranadive SM, Yan H, Weikert M, et al. Vascular dysfunction and physical activity in multiple sclerosis. Med Sci Sports Exerc 2012;44(2):238–43.
18. Mojtahedi MC, Snook EM, Motl RW, et al. Bone health in ambulatory individuals with multiple sclerosis: impact of physical activity, glucocorticoid use, and body composition. J Rehabil Res Dev 2008;45(6):851–61.
19. Ozgocmen S, Bulut S, Ilhan N, et al. Vitamin D deficiency and reduced bone mineral density in multiple sclerosis: effect of ambulatory status and functional capacity. J Bone Miner Metab 2005;23(4):309–13.
20. Marrie RA, Horwitz R, Cutter G, et al. Comorbidity, socioeconomic status and multiple sclerosis. Mult Scler 2008;14(8):1091–8.
21. Marrie RA, Rudick R, Horwitz R, et al. Vascular comorbidity is associated with more rapid disability progression in multiple sclerosis. Neurology 2010;74(13):1041–7.
22. Dishman R, Heath G, Washburn R. Physical activity epidemiology. Champaign (IL): Human Kinetics; 2004.
23. Foster C, Hillsdon M, Thorogood M, et al. Interventions for promoting physical activity. Cochrane Database Syst Rev 2005;(1):CD003180.
24. Warburton DE, Nicol CW, Bredin SS. Health benefits of physical activity: the evidence. CMAJ 2006;174(6):801–9.
25. Tantucci C, Massucci M, Piperno R, et al. Energy cost of exercise in multiple sclerosis patients with low degree of disability. Mult Scler 1996;2(3):161–7.
26. Mostert S, Kesselring J. Effects of a short-term exercise training program on aerobic fitness, fatigue, health perception and activity level of subjects with multiple sclerosis. Mult Scler 2002;8(2):161–8.
27. Brown TR, Kraft GH. Exercise and rehabilitation for individuals with multiple sclerosis. Phys Med Rehabil Clin N Am 2005;16(2):513–55.
28. Armstrong LE, Winant DM, Sawsey PR, et al. Using isokinetic dynamometry to test ambulatory patients with multiple sclerosis. Phys Ther 1983;63(8):1274–9.
29. Lambert CP, Archer RL, Evans WJ. Muscle strength and fatigue during isokinetic exercise in individuals with multiple sclerosis. Med Sci Sports Exerc 2001;33(10):1613–9.
30. Ponichtera JA, Rodgers MM, Glaser RM, et al. Concentric and eccentric isokinetic lower extremity strength in persons with multiple sclerosis. J Orthop Sports Phys Ther 1992;16(3):114–22.
31. Carroll CC, Gallagher PM, Seidle ME, et al. Skeletal muscle characteristics of people with multiple sclerosis. Arch Phys Med Rehabil 2005;86(2):224–9.

32. Ng AV, Miller RG, Gelinas D, et al. Functional relationships of central and peripheral muscle alterations in multiple sclerosis. Muscle Nerve 2004;29(6): 843–52.
33. Kent-Braun JA, Sharma KR, Weiner MW, et al. Effects of exercise on muscle activation and metabolism in multiple sclerosis. Muscle Nerve 1994;17(10): 1162–9.
34. Chen WY, Pierson FM, Burnett CN. Force-time measurements of knee muscle functions of subjects with multiple sclerosis. Phys Ther 1987;67(6):934–40.
35. de Haan A, de Ruiter CJ, van Der Woude LH, et al. Contractile properties and fatigue of quadriceps muscles in multiple sclerosis. Muscle Nerve 2000; 23(10):1534–41.
36. Schwid SR, Thornton CA, Panday S, et al. Quantitative assessment of motor fatigue and strength in MS. Neurology 1999;53(4):743–50.
37. Rice CL, Vollmer TL, Bigland-Ritchie B. Neuromuscular responses of patients with multiple sclerosis. Muscle Nerve 1992;15(10):1123–32.
38. Sharma KR, Kent-Braun J, Mynhier MA, et al. Evidence of an abnormal intramuscular component of fatigue in multiple sclerosis. Muscle Nerve 1995; 18(12):1403–11.
39. Thoumie P, Mevellec E. Relation between walking speed and muscle strength is affected by somatosensory loss in multiple sclerosis. J Neurol Neurosurg Psychiatry 2002;73(3):313–5.
40. Savci S, Inal-Ince D, Arikan H, et al. Six-minute walk distance as a measure of functional exercise capacity in multiple sclerosis. Disabil Rehabil 2005;27(22): 1365–71.
41. Miller A, Dishon S. Health-related quality of life in multiple sclerosis: the impact of disability, gender and employment status. Qual Life Res 2006;15(2):259–71.
42. Olgiati R, Jacquet J, di Prampero PE. Energy cost of walking and exertional dyspnea in multiple sclerosis. Am Rev Respir Dis 1986;134(5):1005–10.
43. Anema JR, Heijenbrok MW, Faes TJ, et al. Cardiovascular autonomic function in multiple sclerosis. J Neurol Sci 1991;104(2):129–34.
44. Pepin EB, Hicks RW, Spencer MK, et al. Pressor response to isometric exercise in patients with multiple sclerosis. Med Sci Sports Exerc 1996;28(6):656–60.
45. Formica CA, Cosman F, Nieves J, et al. Reduced bone mass and fat-free mass in women with multiple sclerosis: effects of ambulatory status and glucocorticoid use. Calcif Tissue Int 1997;61(2):129–33.
46. Lambert CP, Lee Archer R, Evans WJ. Body composition in ambulatory women with multiple sclerosis. Arch Phys Med Rehabil 2002;83(11):1559–61.
47. Hortobagyi T, Dempsey L, Fraser D, et al. Changes in muscle strength, muscle fiber size and myofibrillar gene expression after immobilization and retraining in humans. J Physiol 2000;524(Pt 1):293–304.
48. LaRocca NG, Kalb RC. Efficacy of rehabilitation in multiple sclerosis. Neurorehabil Neural Repair 1992;6(3):147–55.
49. Ponichtera-Mulcare JA. Exercise and multiple sclerosis. Med Sci Sports Exerc 1993;25(4):451–65.
50. Sutherland G, Andersen MD. Exercise and multiple sclerosis: physiological, psychological, and quality of life issues. J Sports Med Phys Fitness 2001; 41(4):421–32.
51. Astrand P, Ekblom B, Messin R, et al. Intra-arterial blood pressure during exercise with different muscle groups. J Appl Physiol 1965;20(2):253–6.
52. Zwiren LD, Bar-Or O. Responses to exercise of paraplegics who differ in conditioning level. Med Sci Sports 1975;7(2):94–8.

53. Schapiro RT, Petajan JH, Kosich D, et al. Role of cardiovascular fitness in multiple sclerosis: a pilot study. Neurorehabil Neural Repair 1988;2(2):43–9.
54. White LJ, Dressendorfer RH. Exercise and multiple sclerosis. Sports Med 2004; 34(15):1077–100.
55. Ponichtera-Mulcare JA, Glaser RM, Mathews T. Maximal aerobic exercise in persons with multiple sclerosis. Clin Kinesiol 1992;46(4):12–21.
56. Sterman AB, Coyle PK, Panasci DJ, et al. Disseminated abnormalities of cardiovascular autonomic functions in multiple sclerosis. Neurology 1985;35(11):1665–8.
57. Petajan JH, Gappmaier E, White AT, et al. Impact of aerobic training on fitness and quality of life in multiple sclerosis. Ann Neurol 1996;39(4):432–41.
58. Iriarte J, de Castro P. Correlation between symptom fatigue and muscular fatigue in multiple sclerosis. Eur J Neurol 1998;5(6):579–85.
59. Latash M, Kalugina E, Nicholas J, et al. Myogenic and central neurogenic factors in fatigue in multiple sclerosis. Mult Scler 1996;1(4):236–41.
60. Mevellec E, Lamotte D, Cantalloube S, et al. Relationship between gait speed and strength parameters in multiple sclerosis [in French]. Ann Readapt Med Phys 2003;46(2):85–90.
61. Uhthoff W. Untersuchungen uber die bei der multiplen herdsklerose vorkommenden augenstorungen. Arch Psychiatr Nervenkr 1889;21:303–420.
62. Petajan JH, White AT. Recommendations for physical activity in patients with multiple sclerosis. Sports Med 1999;27(3):179–91.
63. van Diemen HA, van Dongen MM, Dammers JW, et al. Increased visual impairment after exercise (Uhthoff's phenomenon) in multiple sclerosis: therapeutic possibilities. Eur Neurol 1992;32(4):231–4.
64. Kraft GH, Brown T. Comprehensive management of multiple sclerosis. In: Braddom RL, editor. Physical medicine and rehabilitation. 3rd edition. Philadelphia: Saunders; 2006. p. 1223–42.
65. Saltin B, Hermansen L. Esophageal, rectal, and muscle temperature during exercise. J Appl Physiol 1966;21(6):1757–62.
66. Capello E, Gardella M, Leandri M, et al. Lowering body temperature with a cooling suit as symptomatic treatment for thermosensitive multiple sclerosis patients. Ital J Neurol Sci 1995;16(8):533–9.
67. Kraft G, Alquist A. Effect of microclimate cooling on physical function in multiple sclerosis [abstract]. Mult Scler Clin Lab Res 1996;2(2):114–5.
68. Syndulko K, Woldanski A, Baumhefner R, et al. Preliminary evaluation of lowering tympanic temperature for the symptomatic treatment of multiple sclerosis. Neurorehabil Neural Repair 1995;9(4):205–15.
69. Peterson JL, Bell GW. Aquatic exercise for individuals with multiple sclerosis. Clin Kinesiol 1995;49(3):69–71.
70. Chiara T, Carlos J Jr, Martin D, et al. Cold effect on oxygen uptake, perceived exertion and spasticity in patients with multiple sclerosis. Arch Phys Med Rehabil 1998;79(5):523–8.
71. Motl RW, Gosney JL. Effect of exercise training on quality of life in multiple sclerosis: a meta-analysis. Mult Scler 2008;14(1):129–35.
72. White LJ, McCoy SC, Castellano V, et al. Effect of resistance training on risk of coronary artery disease in women with multiple sclerosis. Scand J Clin Lab Invest 2006;66(4):351–5.
73. DeBolt LS, McCubbin JA. The effects of home-based resistance exercise on balance, power, and mobility in adults with multiple sclerosis. Arch Phys Med Rehabil 2004;85(2):290–7.

74. Gutierrez GM, Chow JW, Tillman MD, et al. Resistance training improves gait kinematics in persons with multiple sclerosis. Arch Phys Med Rehabil 2005; 86(9):1824–9.

75. White LJ, McCoy SC, Castellano V, et al. Resistance training improves strength and functional capacity in persons with multiple sclerosis. Mult Scler 2004;10(6): 668–74.

76. Kasser S, McCubbin JA. Effects of progressive resistance exercise on muscular strength in adults with multiple sclerosis. Med Sci Sports Exerc 1996;28:S143.

77. Kraft G, Alquist A, Lateur B. Effects of resistive exercise on strength in multiple sclerosis (MS). Arch PHys Med Rehabil 1996;77:984.

78. Fisher NM, Leno J, Granger CV, et al. Effects of an anti-fatiguing exercise program on fatigue and physiological function in patients with multiple sclerosis. Neurology 2000;54:A338.

79. Aimeta M, Lampichlera J, Musila U, et al. High and moderate intensities in strength training in multiple sclerosis. Isokinet Exerc Sci 2006;14:153.

80. Taylor NF, Dodd KJ, Prasad D, et al. Progressive resistance exercise for people with multiple sclerosis. Disabil Rehabil 2006;28(18):1119–26.

81. Jones AM, Carter H. The effect of endurance training on parameters of aerobic fitness. Sports Med 2000;29(6):373–86.

82. Carter P, White CM. The effect of general exercise training on effort of walking in patients with multiple sclerosis. 14th International World Confederation for Physical Therapy. Barcelona, June 7–12, 2003; RR-PL-1517.

83. Surakka J, Romberg A, Ruutiainen J, et al. Effects of aerobic and strength exercise on motor fatigue in men and women with multiple sclerosis: a randomized controlled trial. Clin Rehabil 2004;18(7):737–46.

84. Romberg A, Virtanen A, Ruutiainen J, et al. Effects of a 6-month exercise program on patients with multiple sclerosis: a randomized study. Neurology 2004;63(11):2034–8.

85. Romberg A, Virtanen A, Ruutiainen J. Long-term exercise improves functional impairment but not quality of life in multiple sclerosis. J Neurol 2005;252(7): 839–45.

86. Taylor RS. Rehabilitation of persons with multiple sclerosis. In: Braddom RL, editor. Physical medicine and rehabilitation. 2nd edition. Philadelphia: W.B. Saunders; 2000. p. 1117–90.

87. Marrie RA, Horwitz R, Cutter G, et al. The burden of mental comorbidity in multiple sclerosis: frequent, underdiagnosed, and undertreated. Mult Scler 2009; 15(3):385–92.

88. Marrie RA, Horwitz RI, Cutter G, et al. Association between comorbidity and clinical characteristics of MS. Acta Neurol Scand 2011;124(2):135–41.

89. Grahn DA, Murray JV, Heller HC. Cooling via one hand improves physical performance in heat-sensitive individuals with multiple sclerosis: a preliminary study. BMC Neurol 2008;8:14.

90. Mulcare JA. Multiple sclerosis. In: Durstine JL, Moore GE, editors. ACSM's exercise management for persons with chronic diseases and disabilities. Champaign (IL): Human Kinetics; 2003. p. 267–72.

91. Oken BS, Kishiyama S, Zajdel D, et al. Randomized controlled trial of yoga and exercise in multiple sclerosis. Neurology 2004;62(11):2058–64.

92. Madanmohan TD, Balakumar B, Nambinarayanan TK, et al. Effect of yoga training on reaction time, respiratory endurance and muscle strength. Indian J Physiol Pharmacol 1992;36(4):229–33.

93. Morrison EH, Cooper DM, White LJ, et al. Ratings of perceived exertion during aerobic exercise in multiple sclerosis. Arch Phys Med Rehabil 2008;89(8):1570–4.
94. Mazzetti SA, Kraemer WJ, Volek JS, et al. The influence of direct supervision of resistance training on strength performance. Med Sci Sports Exerc 2000;32(6): 1175–84.
95. Kraemer WJ, Adams K, Cafarelli E, et al. American College of Sports Medicine position stand. Progression models in resistance training for healthy adults. Med Sci Sports Exerc 2002;34(2):364–80.
96. White AT. Exercise and MS: challenges and opportunities. Mult Scler Q Rep 2004;23(1):18–20.
97. Jones DA, Rutherford OM, Parker DF. Physiological changes in skeletal muscle as a result of strength training. Q J Exp Physiol 1989;74(3):233–56.

Caregiving in Multiple Sclerosis

Lynda Hillman, DNP, ARNP

KEYWORDS

- Caregiving • Multiple sclerosis • Caregiver burden • Informal care • Disability

KEY POINTS

- Thirty percent of persons with multiple sclerosis (MS) require care because of their disability.
- Eighty percent of MS care is provided by unpaid caregivers.
- Caregiving tasks are time intensive.
- Caregiver burden is common.
- Interventions can reduce caregiver burden and improve caregiver and patient health.

INTRODUCTION

More than 44 million persons in the United States provide informal, unpaid care to their relatives and friends. The value of this informal caregiving is estimated at $375 billion, or twice the cost of formal home care and nursing home care.[1]

Thirty percent of persons with multiple sclerosis (pwMS) require caregiving owing to disability. More than 80% of this care is provided by informal caregivers.[2]

Benefits of Informal Caregiving
- Patient remains in own home and community
- Patient avoids institutionalization
- Patient has familiar caregiver(s)
- Reduced cost to health care system

Caregiver Burden
- Strain on mental and physical health of caregiver
- Loss of employment income due to time demands of caregiving
- Caregiver may lack appropriate training and knowledge

Disclosures: No funding sources or conflict of interest to disclose (L. Hillman).
Multiple Sclerosis Center, University of Washington Medical Center, Box 358815, 1536 North 115th Street, Seattle, WA 98133, USA
E-mail address: lhillman@uw.edu

Phys Med Rehabil Clin N Am 24 (2013) 619–627
http://dx.doi.org/10.1016/j.pmr.2013.06.007

COMPARISON OF CAREGIVING FOR ADULTS WITH MULTIPLE SCLEROSIS AND CAREGIVING FOR OTHER ADULTS

The average adult cared for at home is elderly, and disabled by arthritis, stroke, dementia, or other diseases that tend to occur later in life. By contrast, patients with multiple sclerosis (MS) who require care are young or middle-aged adults. The normal life span is not greatly shortened in MS patients, so impaired function has an earlier onset and longer duration than is found in most other disabled adults.[2] The relapsing, remitting course of the most common form of MS adds uncertainty and complicates care planning (**Table 1**).[3]

ECONOMICS OF MS CAREGIVING

The average value of unpaid caregiving to those with significant disability is an estimated €23,681 (US$30,517) per year.[4] Informal caregiving allows pwMS to avoid institutionalization and to remain in their own home and neighborhoods. More than 40% of pwMS who require care have an annual income of less than $25,000.[5]

Caregiving for a pwMS with an Expanded Disability Status Scale (EDSS) score of 6 to 7 (cane required) ranges from 1.4 to nearly 2 hours per day. Once a patient can no longer ambulate with a cane, the caregiver burden increases dramatically. Care for a pwMS with an EDSS score of 8 to 9 requires 1.7 to 8 hours or more per day.[4] Time spent caregiving for similarly disabled MS patients was reported as the same whether or not the caregiver was in a spousal relationship with the recipient.[3]

CHARACTERISTICS OF MS CAREGIVING TASKS

The variation in task nomenclature between studies limits one's ability to generalize study findings. For example, toileting help may be categorized as personal care, mobility assistance, or activities of daily living (ADLs), depending on the model (**Table 2**).

Carton and colleagues[4] use 4 categories:

- Mobility assistance (transfers, pushing a manual wheelchair, using the toilet)
- Nursing care (giving injections, managing catheter equipment)
- Company (social activities)
- Other (care coordination, gardening)

Table 1
MS caregiving compared with other adult caregiving[2–4]

Caregiver Characteristics	MS Adult	Other Disabled Adult
Gender	47% female	65% female
	53% male	35% male
Age (y)	60	50
Caucasian	90%	73%
Live with care recipient	91%	24%
Spouse/partner of care recipient	62%–78%	20%
Care duties require time taken off work	77%	57%
Duration of care provided (y)	13	4

Table 2
Categories of MS caregiving

Caregiver Tasks	MS Care Recipients[3,6–9] (%)
Meals	50
Hygiene/toileting	45–55
Dressing	69
Ambulation inside the house, transfers	74
Ambulation outside the home	91
ADL caregiving needs	70

O'Hara and colleagues[6] identified 5 major life domains in the care needs of pwMS:

- Personal care (dressing, hygiene, toileting)
- Mobility (ambulation, transfers)
- Household tasks (laundry, cooking)
- Leisure (hobbies, social activities)
- Employment (paid occupation)

Pakenham[7] classified MS caregiving tasks into 4 categories:

- ADLs (toileting, feeding, dressing)
- Instrumental ADLs (shopping, transportation, housework)
- Psychoemotional (management of fatigue, dealing with cognitive difficulties)
- Sociopractical (managing finances, assisting with exercise).

Tasks such as transfers, in-home ambulation, and toileting may not take up much time per occurrence, but frequency results in significant total time.

CAREGIVER BURDEN

Caregiving burden may be objective (the visible and easily quantifiable demands on caregiver time) or subjective (the emotional strain as perceived by the caregiver).[10] More than 20% of MS caregivers experience caregiver burden.[8,11] Moreover, caregiver burden may be underreported.

Caregiver burden is mediated[12] by:

- Disease severity
- Presence or absence of formal and informal support networks
- Participation in respite and other non-caregiver activities
- Presence of other or conflicting roles

Problem Areas Reported by Caregivers[3,5,7,13,14]

- Physical strain of caring for mobility-impaired patients
- Constant unrelenting nature of care needs
- Sleep interruptions due to caregiving tasks
- Quality of relationship with pwMS
- Restrictions from caregiving
- Lack of knowledge about MS
- Lack of necessary assistive equipment
- Own aging and own health problems

The negative impact of caregiving may cause physical, mental, social, and financial strain.[13] The unpredictable nature of MS may exacerbate caregiver stress.[15]

Increased caregiver stress has been associated with increased time spent on caregiving.[7] However, increased time and duration of caregiving has also been found to be associated with increased caregiver satisfaction and benefit finding.[10,16]

At-home respite services are used by only 5% of MS caregivers. Adult daycare services are used by only 3.6%.[5] It is not clear whether lack of use is due to lack of awareness, rejection of outside help, or lack of access to services owing to financial or geographic limitations.

Subjective caregiver stress does not relate to degree of caregiver self-efficacy.[15] Studies on gender in relation to subject caregiver stress have contradictory findings.[14] However, female caregivers report increased objective caregiver burden in comparison with male caregivers.[6]

Caregiving has an adverse effect on the ability of caregivers to continue paid employment.[3]

- Fifty-one percent reduced their employment hours as a result of caregiver responsibilities within the last year.
- Thirty-six percent expected to reduce their employment hours during the next year.

Caregiving may have a negative impact on the health of the caregiver (**Table 3**).

Depression in the pwMS can increase the likelihood of emotional distress in the caregiver.[12] This problem is a significant one, as 50% to 75% of pwMS are estimated to have depression.[12,14]

Impaired cognition, irritability, apathy, agitation, delusions, and disinhibition were associated with high levels of caregiver distress and reduced caregiver quality of life. Higher levels of physical deficits were related to higher caregiver distress, but not to caregiver quality of life.[12]

Many MS caregivers (25%–55%)[5,17] believe they would benefit from mental health counseling. However, only 35% of those who reported a need for counseling actually sought treatment.[5] The primary reason (60%) for not seeking mental health counseling was financial constraints such as high copays, or lack of insurance coverage.

The unmet needs for resources and information reported by caregivers are extensive (**Table 4**).

CAREGIVING BENEFIT

Most caregivers report a sense of satisfaction with the caregiving role (**Table 5**).[16]

Factors Associated with Increased Caregiver Benefit[16,17]
- Older age
- Lower level of caregiver education

Table 3 Negative impact on caregiver health	
Common Caregiver Health Complaints	**Reported by Ref.[8] (%)**
Anxiety	85
Fatigue	82
Back pain	68
Insomnia	74
Impaired sex and impaired spousal relationship	75
Sadness/depression	77

Table 4
Unmet resource and information needs reported by caregivers

Resource Needs	Caregivers Reporting[5,17] (%)
Mobility device (for pwMS)	85
Access to services (navigating insurance, hiring home help)	75
Home modifications	62
Support group (for pwMS)	33
Home modifications and assistive technology	29.8
Support group (for caregivers)	28
Appropriate transportation to medical care	24
Information Needs	**Caregivers Reporting[3,17] (%)**
Coping with caregiving, caregiving/life balance	50
Physical aspects of MS	49
Transfer techniques	47
Patient safety at home	40
Toileting and incontinence	33
Communications with MS health providers	20
Managing own health	20
Planning for future (long-term care, retirement planning)	21
Understanding MS (disease course, medications, side effects)	19.9

- Lower perception of emotional drain
- Longer hours of caregiving
- Longer duration of caregiving

Factors Associated with Decreased Caregiver Benefit[16]
- Spousal relationship
- Higher level of caregiver education

The lower level of caregiver benefit seen in caregiver spouses is likely due to diminished or lost role of the spouse. Those with higher education may see more opportunity lost when caregiving restricts employment options.[16]

Pakenham and Cox[18] developed the 18-item Benefit-Finding in MS Care (BFiMS-Care) scale through a longitudinal study, which measures benefit finding.

BFiMSCare Domains
- Enriched relationship (with pwMS)
- Inspiration (facing disability with resilience)
- Family relationship growth (with other relatives)
- Other relationship opportunities (medical providers, support groups)

Table 5
Caregiver satisfaction

Statement	Agreement (%) Most or Always
Caregiving is rewarding	66
Proud of care provided	80
Caregiving gives sense of accomplishment	57

- Spiritual ("God's will")
- Lifestyle/health (reason to improve own health)

Increased benefit finding was associated with higher rates of adjustment to the MS diagnosis in the pwMS. However, the reverse was not found; that is, a higher levels of distress in the pwMS was not associated with a low level of benefit finding by the caregiver.[18]

Low benefit finding was most often found to be associated with a spousal relationship, similar to the findings of the study of caregiver satisfaction by Buchanan and Huang.[16] Men were more likely than women to report lower scores in the domains of inspiration, family relationship, other relationship opportunities, spirituality, and lifestyle.[10]

Coping Strategies by Caregivers

Caregivers may use reframing techniques to "make sense" of the MS caregiving reality.[19] Stressors are then redefined into more beneficial terms. The benefits may include gains in insight, personal growth, or sense of reward at being needed by the pwMS.

Common Sense-Making Themes[19]
- Catalyst for change (opportunity for growth)
- Relationship with pwMS (closeness through adversity)
- Incomprehensibility (cannot make sense of MS; random fate)
- Attribution of cause of MS (heredity, pwMS behavior)
- Spiritual (God's will)
- Acceptance (adjustment)

Female caregivers were more likely than their male counterparts to consider the caregiving experience an opportunity for positive change or spiritual growth. This finding may arise from societal expectations of women's role as caregivers.

Caregivers who were unable to continue paid employment were more apt to consider MS caregiving as "incomprehensible" than caregivers who had not lost employment. Perhaps the financial and personal impact from job loss was too severe to allow easy redefinition.

Benefit-finding and sense-making strategies may appear promising as cognitive restructuring interventions; however, to date there is little evidence of their efficacy.[19] Nevertheless, the rehabilitation medicine professional should be familiar with their use by patients.

ASSESSMENT OF CAREGIVER BURDEN

Open-ended questioning of the caregiver will provide useful information on caregiving responsibilities, burden of stressors, and self-care habits. A caring manner and brief discussion of the caregiving burden and reward concepts will help to minimize possible caregiver guilt that may interfere with acknowledgment of burden. Most caregivers will be pleased at the opportunity to discuss caregiving.

When use of a formal assessment tool is desirable, the Zarit Burden Interview,[20] a self-administered questionnaire that can be completed within 10 minutes, has been often used with MS caregivers.[21,22]

INTERVENTIONS TO IMPROVE CAREGIVER HEALTH AND REDUCE BURDEN

Interventions to decrease objective caregiver burden, such as need for mobility equipment, are relatively straightforward. Interventions to decrease subjective caregiver

Table 6
Rehabilitation therapy/consult interventions

Referral	Benefits
Physical therapy/Occupational therapy	Evaluation of home environment Assistive equipment for mobility, activities of daily life Teaching of transfer techniques Home exercise program to increase/maintain function
Speech therapy	Cognitive rehabilitation Compensatory strategies for patient and caregiver
Psychology	Counseling for coping strategies, stress reduction Psychotherapy for depression, anxiety
Neuropsychology/Detailed cognitive evaluation	Identify need for cognitively related job accommodations
Assistive technology	Adapted computer use
Orthotics	Braces to improve mobility and positioning
Social work	Information on respite care, benefit eligibility at state or national level
Rehabilitation/Occupational counseling	Job accommodation counseling, disability benefits counseling
Psychiatry	Medication consult, management of mental health issues

burden are far more challenging. At present there is no clear agreement on the most effective interventions for reducing caregiver strain, which manifests as anxiety, insomnia, poor health, and related less tangible effects.[15]

Any cognitive restructuring techniques should be presented carefully, so as not to be seen as unrealistic or a minimalization of the severe impact of MS.[18] Interventions that improve the dyadic relationship of caregiver and pwMS are associated with increased benefit finding.[8]

Female caregivers may gain benefit from internal home space made over for their exclusive use as an area of respite. Women are more accepting of help from support systems such as friends, relatives, and health care professionals than are men.[15]

Opportunities at Office Visits to Decrease Caregiver Burden[22]
- Talk with caregiver as well as with patient
- Validate importance of caregiving
- Provide clear, simplified information on medical care
- Encourage self-care: health diet, moderate exercise, and enrichment activity
- Recommend respite services
- Inform about community programs and support groups
- Encourage increased social participation

Many common rehabilitation therapies are useful interventions that improve the health of caregivers and decrease the burden of caregiving.[2] Interprofessional collaboration also helps meet caregiver needs for information and support (**Table 6**).

SUMMARY

More than 30% of MS patients receive caregiving services from unpaid, informal caregivers, usually a spouse or other relative. Time spent on caregiving increases significantly with severity of disability. Persons with advanced MS may require 8 to 12 hours of caregiving per day. Caregivers of pwMS often find benefits of personal growth and insight through caregiving. Caregiving may also take a physical and emotional toll on the caregiver, and cause reduced earning potential and poorer health. Caregivers report significant needs for support, information, and assistive devices to help ease the caregiving burden. Rehabilitation medicine professionals are uniquely positioned to identify needs and manage interventions to reduce the burden on caregivers.

REFERENCES

1. National Alliance for Caregiving in collaboration with AARP. Caregiving in the U.S. A focused look at those caring for someone age 50 or older. Available at: http://www.caregiving.org/data/FINALRegularExSum50plus.pdf. Accessed January 20, 2013.
2. Beer S, Khan F, Kesselring J. Rehabilitation interventions in multiple sclerosis: an overview. J Neurol 2012;259(9):1994–2008.
3. Buchanan RJ, Radin D, Chakravorty BJ, et al. Informal care giving to more disabled people with multiple sclerosis. Disabil Rehabil 2009;31(15):1244–56.
4. Carton H, Loos R, Pacolet J, et al. A quantitative study of unpaid caregiving in multiple sclerosis. Mult Scler 2000;6:274–9.
5. Buchanan RJ, Radin D, Chakravorty BJ, et al. Perceptions of informal care givers: health and support services provided to people with multiple sclerosis. Disabil Rehabil 2010;32(6):500–10.
6. O'Hara L, de Souza L, Ide L. The nature of care giving in a community sample of people with multiple sclerosis. Disabil Rehabil 2004;26(24):1401–10.
7. Pakenham KI. The nature of caregiving in multiple sclerosis: development of the caregiving tasks in multiple sclerosis scale. Mult Scler 2007;13(7):929–38.
8. Forbes A, While A, Mathes L. Informal carer activities, carer burden and health status in multiple sclerosis. Clin Rehabil 2007;21(6):563–75.
9. Minden SL, Frankel D, Hadden L, et al. The Sonya Slifka longitudinal multiple sclerosis study: methods and sample characteristics. Mult Scler 2006;12:24–36.
10. Pakenham KI. The positive impact of multiple sclerosis (MS) on carers: associations between carer benefit finding and positive and negative adjustment domains. Disabil Rehabil 2005;27(17):985–97.
11. Buchanan RJ, Radin D, Huang C. Burden among male caregivers assisting people with multiple sclerosis. Gend Med 2010;7(6):637–46.
12. Figved N, Myhr KM, Larsen JP, et al. Caregiver burden in multiple sclerosis: the impact of neuropsychiatric symptoms. J Neurol Neurosurg Psychiatry 2007;78(10):1097–102.
13. Finlayson M, Cho C. A descriptive profile of caregivers of older adults with MS and the assistance they provide. Disabil Rehabil 2008;30(24):1848–57.
14. McKeown LP, Porter-Armstrong AP, Baxter GD. The needs and experiences of caregivers of individuals with multiple sclerosis: a systematic review. Clin Rehabil 2003;17:234–48.
15. Khan F, Pallant J, Brand C. Caregiver strain and factors associated with caregiver self-efficacy and quality of life in a community cohort with multiple sclerosis. Disabil Rehabil 2007;29(16):1241–50.
16. Buchanan RJ, Huang C. Caregiver perceptions of accomplishment from assisting people with multiple sclerosis. Disabil Rehabil 2010;34(1):53–61.

17. Finlayson M, Garcia JD, Preissner K. Development of an educational programme for caregivers of people aging with multiple sclerosis. Occup Ther Int 2008;15(1): 4–17.

18. Pakenham KI, Cox S. Development of the benefit finding in multiple sclerosis caregiving scale: a longitudinal study of relations between benefit finding and adjustment. Br J Health Psychol 2008;13:583–602.

19. Pakenham KI. Making sense of caregiving for persons with multiple sclerosis (MS): the dimensional structure of sense making and relations with positive and negative adjustment. Int J Behav Med 2008;15(3):241–52.

20. Zarit SH, Reever KE, Bach-Peterson J. Relatives of the impaired elderly: correlates of feelings of burden. Gerontologist 1980;20(6):649–55.

21. Rivera-Navarro J, Benito-Leon J, Oreja-Guevara C, et al. Burden and health-related quality of life of Spanish caregivers of persons with multiple sclerosis. Mult Scler 2009;15(11):1347–55.

22. Buhse M. Assessment of caregiver burden in families of persons with multiple sclerosis. J Neurosci Nurs 2008;40(1):25–31.

Activities of Daily Living
Evaluation and Treatment in Persons with Multiple Sclerosis

Ann Buzaid, MA, OTR/L, ATP[a],*, Mary Pat Dodge, MS, OTR/L[a],
Lynne Handmacher, OTR/L[b], Pamela J. Kiltz, MOTR/L[a]

KEYWORDS

- Activities of daily living • ADL • Multiple sclerosis • Occupational therapy
- Adaptive equipment • Home safety

KEY POINTS

- Common symptoms and impairments of multiple sclerosis can create significant deficits in activities of daily living, which can be addressed through evaluation and treatment by the occupational therapist.
- For a person with multiple sclerosis, adaptive equipment is often recommended and necessary for safety and independence during activities of daily living and functional transfers.
- Safety issues and functional impairments in a person with multiple sclerosis indicate the need for a referral to an occupational therapist.

INTRODUCTION

This article describes the types of activities of daily living (ADLs), assessment, treatment and training strategies, and adaptive equipment that are used with persons who have multiple sclerosis (MS). Because MS affects the central nervous system, it can result in both cognitive and physical changes, which affect the person's function along a continuum of mild to very severe limitation. Limitations can affect single or multiple areas and include impaired vision, cognitive deficits, fatigue, impaired coordination, muscle weakness, and spasticity. Along with the broad spectrum of potential impairment, each individual brings their own abilities, priorities, resources, and unique style of performing ADLs.

Disclosures: The authors have no funding sources or conflicts of interest to disclose.
[a] Department of Occupational Therapy, University of Washington Medical Center, Box 356154, Seattle, WA 98195, USA; [b] Private Practice, 4728 Silver Bow Road Northeast, Tacoma, WA 98422, USA
* Corresponding author.
E-mail address: abuzaid@u.washington.edu

ADLS

It is typically the role of the occupational therapist to address the evaluation and treatment of deficits in the area of ADLs. ADLs are generally grouped into 2 categories:

1. Basic ADLs (BADLs) also called personal ADLs (PADLs) are those things we do that are considered fundamental to taking care of ourselves.
2. Instrumental ADLs (IADLs) are those activities that may affect our ability to live on our own but are not necessary for personal daily functioning.

The American Occupational Therapy Association (AOTA) defines 12 BADLs and 11 IADLs[1]:

BADLs/PADLs
- Bathing and showering
- Bowel and bladder management
- Dressing
- Feeding
- Functional mobility
- Personal device care, such as care for dentures or hearing aids
- Personal hygiene and grooming
- Sexual activity
- Toilet hygiene

IADLs
- Care of others
- Care of pets
- Child rearing
- Communication management
- Community mobility, including driving
- Financial management
- Health management and maintenance
- Meal preparation and clean-up
- Religious observations
- Safety procedures and emergency responses
- Shopping

Occupational therapists work as part of a team, which may include nurses, physical therapists, physicians, psychologists, recreational therapists, speech and language pathologists, and vocational counselors. Depending on the team and the setting, occupational therapists may be primarily responsible for evaluating and providing treatment and training for most of the ADLs. However, for some deficits in ADLs, responsibility for evaluation and treatment may be shared with other disciplines. For example, bowel and bladder management are frequently assessed and taught by nursing; however, occupational therapists may train in or adapt equipment to develop the person's independence.

ADAPTIVE DEVICES

Occupational therapists frequently recommend adaptive equipment, assistive devices, and splints or other positioning devices to aid persons with MS in completing their ADLs. It is most beneficial that the individual be given the opportunity to trial the equipment during treatment sessions to ensure that the equipment is not only physically usable but also cognitively and emotionally acceptable to the person.

Some persons with MS are more readily able to see adaptive equipment as a useful tool than others.

Adaptive devices specific to cognitive impairment:

- Daily planners/calendars
- Checklists/to-do lists
- Medication sets
- Electronic devices: smart phones, tablets, alarms

Adaptive devices specific to home safety and ADLs:

- Personal medical alarms
- Bathroom equipment (grab bars, raised toilet seats/commodes, bath/shower seats)
- Mobility equipment (wheelchairs, walkers, canes, floor/ceiling lifts, stair lifts)
- Dressing equipment (reachers, sock aids, shoe horns, elastic laces, button hooks)
- Eating devices (large-handled utensils, rocker knife, u-cuff, lip plate)
- Grooming devices
- Toileting devices
- Bathing devices
- Kitchen/cooking devices

EVALUATION OF ADLS

The occupational therapist performs a comprehensive evaluation of persons with MS, including strength testing, measurement of range of motion, fine and gross motor assessment, vision screening, sensation, and cognition. ADLs are assessed through interview and performance of the activity. Activities are typically scored by the level of assistance that the person requires to complete the activities. An example of a functional measure is the Functional Independence Measure (FIM). Once the evaluation is complete, the occupational therapist and the person with MS devise treatment goals tailored to improve function in the areas of deficit and importance to the individual. For example, a person with MS may be unable to dress herself. She may choose to have her husband put on her socks but may want to work on becoming independent in putting on her brassiere and shirt (**Table 1**).

IMPAIRMENTS RELATED TO MOVEMENT

Persons with MS may have 1 or more impairments affecting movement, including weakness, spasticity, tremors, and incoordination. These symptoms subsequently affect performance of BADLs and IADLs. Occupational therapists can help assess, treat, and make recommendations based on the severity of the symptoms listed earlier.

ASSESSMENT

Self-care assessments often begin with determining the level and quality of a person's movements. Once this key area is assessed, it helps the therapist visualize the individual at home and on a typical day.

Important areas to assess related to impairments of movement:

1. How does the person move through space (ie, use of power or manual wheelchair vs assistive device during ambulation vs independence with ambulation)? Are they able to stand or push up from the wheelchair for even short periods?

Table 1
FIM measure developed and trademarked by Uniform Data System for Medical Rehabilitation, a division of UB Foundation Activities

FIM Scoring Criteria	
Score	**Description**
No helper required	
7	Complete independence
6	Modified independence (patient requires use of a device, but no physical assistance)
Helper (modified dependence)	
5	Supervision or set-up
4	Minimal contact assistance (patient can perform $\geq$75% or more of task)
3	Moderate assistance (patient can perform 50%–74% of task)
Helper (complete dependence)	
2	Maximal assistance (patient can perform 25%–49% of task)
1	Total assistance (patient can perform <25% of the task or requires >1 person to assist)
0	Activity does not occur

2. If nonambulatory, how does the person transfer from 1 surface to another (ie, from the wheelchair to and from the toilet)?
3. If ambulatory, does the person safely bend down, negotiate a walker in doorways, and use outside supports for stability when reaching or rising from a sitting position?
4. What position can the person safely assume while getting dressed, groomed, or washed?
5. If using a wheelchair, can the individual access the bathroom, kitchen, bedroom, and other living spaces?
6. To what extent can the person reach for, move, and handle objects?

These variables determine which assistive devices and compensatory strategies might be used to make daily living tasks less difficult.

TREATMENT STRATEGIES

One of the roles of the occupational therapist when treating persons with MS is to help manage symptoms to maximize independence and safety with ADLs. Home modifications are often recommended in order for a primary wheelchair user, for example, to access the bathroom, enter/exit the home, or retrieve needed items from high and low spaces. Equipment recommendations are also an important part of the occupational therapy process and are based on how the person can perform or be most safely assisted with a functional transfer.

Transfer Training and Equipment

A functional transfer may include getting in and out of bed, on and off the toilet/commode, and in and out of the shower. A primary wheelchair user with significant extensor spasms in the hips and lower extremities, for example, is at risk for falls in the bathroom during transfers, because these types of spasms typically bring the hips and pelvis anteriorly out of the wheelchair. Persons with MS who have this type of spasticity often need to remain in a seated position to get out of the wheelchair and into a tub/shower combination. A tub transfer bench is recommended for several reasons, including:

1. It allows the person to maintain a hips-flexed, knees-flexed, and ankles-dorsiflexed position, which inhibits extensor spasms.
2. It allows the person to enter/exit the tub without standing to step over the tub ledge.
3. It allows the person to remain seated for bathing.

Mobilizing and Reaching for Dressing

Threading feet through pant legs (as in lower body dressing and managing clothing up and down over hips) and toileting are some of the most physically taxing self-care tasks for the person with MS, or they may be unable to perform them because of weakness. The individual may not have enough strength to rise to a standing position to get pants up over the hips, so the occupational therapist may suggest clothing modifications or getting dressed from bed level. Rolling back and forth in bed may improve ease with which the person or a caregiver can help pull pants up. Some persons with MS can also use the functions of a hospital bed (head and foot of bed raised) to better reach their feet in a supported position. Adaptive devices such as reachers and dressing sticks can compensate for limited ability to reach the feet during dressing. Adaptive techniques may also be taught for the person with hemiplegia.

Preparatory Methods Training

Teaching preparatory methods can effect changes in a person's ability to perform self care tasks most independently. These methods include stretching and range-of-motion programs, appropriate strengthening exercises, splinting, and timing treatments to maximize muscle function after chemodenervation or baclofen trials.

SENSORY-RELATED SYMPTOMS
Impaired Vision

Impaired vision is often the first symptom of MS. Visual deficits may be the result of optic neuritis, diplopia, or nystagmus. Diplopia and nystagmus can cause impaired balance. The symptoms of optic neuritis that are most likely to continue are impaired color and contrast perception. Heat, exercise, and fever can exacerbate the symptoms. Frequently, visual deficits resolve or are addressed by an ophthalmologist. If the visual deficits affect self-care tasks, occupational therapy can assist with adaptive techniques and equipment to help compensate. Fall prevention, safety, and independence are areas that occupational therapy can address.

Assessment

Persons with MS are frequently diagnosed with a visual deficit before the referral to occupational therapy; however, if a visual deficit is suspected, an assessment can include a quick visual screen, with subsequent referral back to the physician for more specific diagnosis. Further assessment related to vision may include:

- Determining the person's particular areas of difficulty in BADLs and IADLs
- Completing a kitchen evaluation for safety
- Completing a driving evaluation by an adaptive driving specialist

Treatment

Persons with MS are taught compensatory techniques to complete ADLs safely.

1. There are multiple adaptations for impaired contrast vision. For example, a white plate placed on a dark placemat makes the plate easier to see. Computer settings can be changed: black lettering on a yellow background may be easier to see; stickers with large print letters in a variety of contrast patterns can be applied to the keyboard keys.
2. Persons with MS are helped with organization for home and work to help them be more efficient, safer, and less frustrated. For example, food items can be organized with the more frequently used items toward the front of the refrigerator shelf or grouped with items that are used together.
3. Persons with MS are assisted to obtain adaptive equipment. For example, voice recognition software for computers eliminates the need to see the keyboard. There are many styles of magnifiers; the person is assisted to choose the most suitable one given their particular activities and needs.
4. Safety is addressed. For example, a person may be directed to decrease glare, improve task-specific lighting, or eliminate busy background patterns. Bathroom and kitchen safety are of particular concern. If balance is a concern, sitting to bathe may be safer. Elimination of throw rugs helps prevent tripping. Safety with cutting foods may entail using a specialized cutting board. Persons with MS are taught awareness and compensatory techniques to deal with impaired vision when moving about in their environment.

PAIN

Pain can be musculoskeletal or neurologic. Occupational therapists often address musculoskeletal causes of pain as well as spasticity.

Assessment

Persons with MS are asked to rate their pain at rest and when performing functional activities. The impact of the pain on ADLs is explored. Strength and range of motion in the upper extremities is tested. The person's functional mobility for bed, toilet, shower/bath, and car transfers is assessed. If the person is in a wheelchair, their positioning in the chair is evaluated. The extent of spasticity in the upper extremities, trunk, and pelvis is assessed.

Typical treatment includes:

- Exercise training, including aerobic, stretching, and range of motion.
- Assistance with adaptive devices and techniques. For example, equipment such as reachers and sock aids may decrease strain on the back when dressing.
- Training for proper positioning and methods of changing positions both in bed and in the wheelchair.
- Splinting in the upper extremity. Splinting is particularly beneficial with instances of spasticity to prevent painful contractures and postures.
- Training in relaxation techniques.

IMPAIRED SENSATION

A typical symptom of MS is paresthesia. Persons with MS may describe it as numbness, tingling, pins and needles, burning, or itching.

Assessment

The impact of impaired sensation on ADLs is explored with the person with MS. For example, is numbness causing loss of balance or dropping of items or is the pins-and-needles sensation interrupting sleep?

Treatment Examples

- A person with numbness is trained to use their vision to compensate when carrying a cup of coffee to prevent dropping it. Using a commuter cup prevents spilling.
- If persons with MS have loss of balance from numbness in the lower extremities, they are trained to sit to dress and bathe for safety.
- Desensitization therapy may help decrease the discomfort from paresthesia.

COGNITIVE IMPAIRMENT

According to the National Multiple Sclerosis Society (NMSS), approximately 50% of persons with MS develop problems with cognition and 5% to 10% develop problems severe enough to significantly interfere with ADLs.[2]

The AOTA defines cognition as "information-processing functions performed by the brain that include attention, memory, executive functions (ie, planning, problem solving, self-monitoring, self-awareness), comprehension and formation of speech, calculation ability, visual perception, and praxis skills (motor planning)."[3]

In general, persons with MS often have deficits in the areas of memory, divided attention, information processing, executive functions, visual perception, and word-finding. Typically, general intellect, long-term memory, conversational skills, and reading comprehension remain intact.[2]

Other interesting statements from the NMSS[2]:

1. Cognitive function correlates with the number of lesions and lesion areas on magnetic resonance imaging, as well as brain atrophy.
2. Cognitive impairment is not related to physical limitations. A person with almost no physical limitation can have significant cognitive impairment, whereas a person who is disabled physically can be unaffected cognitively.
3. Cognitive changes generally progress slowly but are unlikely to improve dramatically once they have begun.
4. Although cognitive changes are more common later in the disease, they can occur at any time and may even be a first symptom of MS.
5. Certain aspects of MS can decrease cognitive functioning, such as fatigue, medications, stress, depression, and being in an exacerbation.
6. Early recognition, assessment, and treatment of cognitive function are important, because these changes (along with fatigue) can significantly affect a person's quality of life and are the primary cause of early departure from the workforce.

Even subtle cognitive impairments can influence many areas of an individual's life, including social participation, subjective well-being, education, employment, and functional performance of ADLs.

Assessment

Cognition is an important area of assessment when evaluating functional performance of ADLs. One of the key factors to determine is the person's level of self-awareness of disease-related deficits. Lack of awareness of cognitive deficits significantly impairs judgment for making decisions and restricts the person's ability to learn compensatory strategies. For example, if a person is not aware that they are forgetting appointments or forgetting to take their medications, using checklists and calendars or a medication set to assist with memory deficits is not acknowledged by the patient as a needed strategy.

Another key factor to evaluate is the overall concept of home safety.

Important areas to assess related to cognition and safety:

1. Is the person living alone? The level of support from others is crucial when looking at cognitive deficits. A person living alone has higher responsibilities, such as managing finances, shopping for and preparing meals, maintaining a clean and safe environment, and obtaining transportation.
2. Is the person able to independently manage medications?
3. Is the person independently initiating personal self-care, such as grooming, eating, and bathing?
4. Is the person able to manage their bowel and bladder and solve issues with incontinence?
5. Is the person safe to be driving?
6. Is the person experiencing falls?
7. Is the person able to learn new information or carry out doctors' instructions?

Cognitive deficits such as those listed earlier can have a significant effect on the patient's abilities to perform both BADLs and IADLs.

One typical area for concern with ADL performance and cognitive deficits is the ability to solve problems in the setting of declining physical abilities. For example, a patient with MS may develop lack of trunk control or hand control that makes it too difficult to bend down and reach their feet for donning shoes and socks as they have always done. A patient with no cognitive deficits tends to figure out another way to safely reach their feet and get the job done. A person with lack of executive functions is not able to trial alternative methods and often gives up the activity that is too difficult (eg, by wearing slip-on shoes/sandals and no socks).

Another area of concern with ADL performance and cognitive deficits is poor judgment and poor decision making. For example, persons with MS who have decreased awareness of deficits often overestimate their abilities to perform a familiar activity, such as getting up to use the toilet at night. They may not take the time to fully awaken and turn on a light or may not take issues of urinary urgency into account. As a result, they are at risk for falling.

Lack of memory and lack of ability to divide attention can also cause safety issues, such as forgetting a pan on the stovetop because the patient left the kitchen to answer the phone.

Treatment Strategies

Once the areas of cognitive deficits are identified, the first strategy for training is to help bring awareness of deficits to the person to teach compensatory strategies. This process may require feedback from multiple sources other than the therapist and often requires involvement of family members to support the plan of care.

Problem-Solving Assistance

Identifying specific areas of problems with performance of ADLs and assisting in problem solving can be a concrete way to improve safety and performance for the person with MS. For example, for the person who has not been able to don their shoes and socks, the occupational therapist can trial various positions or devices to allow them to return to independence with this activity. They can then carry over performance of the activity to the home setting. This strategy is particularly helpful when an adaptive device is needed. Use of a device makes a common activity unfamiliar and more difficult to learn for a person with cognitive impairment.

Another example of assisting with problem solving may be how to safely manage meal preparation for the person who lives alone. This assistance could mean teaching a more impaired patient to cook only with a microwave oven, or it could mean introducing the patient with hand weakness to an adaptive sharp knife that is safer to use.

Developing a Structured Daily Routine

Another treatment strategy for the person with MS who is cognitively impaired is developing a structured daily routine. Writing down a daily schedule, which includes important daily functions such as taking medications, completing home exercises, meals, and other self-care tasks, is a compensatory strategy that allows the person to control and track the day. Creating a basic structure is trialed during therapy sessions. The person must establish the habit of creating their own daily plan each morning or evening to allow for day-to-day changes, such as doctor or social appointments. A similar compensatory strategy involves creating checklists and to-do lists. A checklist can address a specific situation, such as "What do I need to do and take before I leave the house?" A to-do list allows management of important tasks that may take days or weeks to complete.

Caregiver Training

Another important area addressed during occupational therapy treatment is training of caregivers or family members. Caregivers need to know the level of supervision required during performance of ADLs so that the patient is as independent as possible but still safe. For example, instead of the caregiver telling the person what will be happening next in the day, the caregiver can remind or refer the person to their daily plan. This point is also relevant for activities that require physical assistance. The caregiver is trained to provide the least amount of assistance needed to avoid having the person tune out and become dependent. This strategy allows the person with MS to have as many opportunities as possible to stay active both cognitively and physically.

FATIGUE

Fatigue is among the most common and debilitating symptoms of MS, affecting approximately 80% of persons who have the disease. (See the article by Cook and colleagues elsewhere in this issue for further exploration of this topic.) MS fatigue can interfere with one's ability to maintain employment and complete ADLs/IADLs. An occupational therapist can help a person with MS manage fatigue through energy-conservation techniques and pacing.

Assessment

Assessment can take several forms:

- Information can come from self-reporting by the person with MS as well as gathering input from family and friends.
- The person with MS may be asked to keep daily and weekly logs.
- The therapist may take the patient step by step through a typical day, having the person with MS give an example of the activities that occur on an hour-by-hour basis.

- The person with MS may be asked to rate their fatigue on a scale like the pain rating scale of 0 to 10. This strategy is useful to show progress after training.
- There are also several standard fatigue questionnaires that the therapist can use.

Treatment Strategies

Training in energy conservation and pacing go hand in hand. Energy-conservation training encompasses the use of adaptive techniques/work simplification, and adaptive devices and equipment. Pacing training looks at spreading activities throughout the day, week, or month in a manner that eases fatigue.

Examples of pacing and energy conservation:

- Preparatory work for the evening meal can be started in the morning, when energy is good, then a few quick tasks can be performed to finish the meal at dinner time, when fatigue is greater (pacing). Persons with MS can use a food processer to chop foods instead of doing it by hand. They can sit at a table or low counter to do preparatory work instead of standing (energy conservation).
- Bathing, dressing, grooming, and fixing breakfast in the morning before work are too much for persons with MS who have fatigue. Instead, they could shower at night before going to bed. Sitting during dressing and grooming saves energy, as does using a reacher to help put on pants if leaning down is difficult. Nonperishable breakfast items can be set out the night before.

SUMMARY

MS symptoms can create mild to severe changes in a person's abilities to perform ADLs. Even a mild impairment of abilities to carry out ADLs can have a significant impact on quality of life in persons with MS.

This article described:

- The specific nature of ADLs in relationship to common MS symptoms and impairments
- The role of the occupational therapist in assessing and treating ADL impairments in persons with MS
- Signs of safety issues and impairments to function that indicate the need for a referral to an occupational therapist
- Treatment strategies and adaptive equipment used to maximize the patient's level of independence and safety in the environment

REFERENCES

1. American Occupational Therapy Association (AOTA). 2013. Available at: http://aota.org/Consumers.aspx. Accessed January 13, 2013.
2. National Multiple Sclerosis Society (NMSS). 2013. About MS>what we know about MS>Symptoms>cognitive dysfunction. Available at: http://www.nationalmssociety.org. Accessed February 16, 2013.
3. American Occupational Therapy Association (AOTA). 2013. Cognition, cognitive rehabilitation, and occupational performance. Available at: http://www.aota.org/Practitioners/Official/Statements/Advance-prepublication. Accessed February 16, 2013.

Movement Disorders in Multiple Sclerosis

Patricia K. Oakes, MD, JD[a], Sindhu R. Srivatsal, MD, MPH[a],
Marie Y. Davis, MD, PhD[a], Ali Samii, MD[b],*

KEYWORDS

• Multiple sclerosis • Movement disorder • Tremor • Ataxia • Restless legs

KEY POINTS

- Tremor, ataxia, and restless legs are the most common movement disorders in multiple sclerosis.
- Treatment of movement disorders in multiple sclerosis is generally similar to their treatment in patients without multiple sclerosis.
- The long-term efficacy of deep brain stimulation for treatment of tremor has not been well established.
- Injections of botulinum toxin are effective in treating focal dystonias and hemifacial spasm.

INTRODUCTION

Movement disorders constitutes a subspecialty of neurology focusing on a variety of conditions characterized by hypokinetic, hyperkinetic, or abnormally coordinated movements,[1] which include tremor, dystonia, parkinsonism, myoclonus, chorea, ballismus, tics, restless limbs, and ataxia, among others. The term "movement disorders" may be used to refer to either abnormal movements or syndromes that cause such abnormal movements. The classification of movement disorders is based on phenomenology, individual syndromes, or etiology.[2] This article reviews the terminology used to describe movement disorders, discusses individual movement disorders and their occurrence in patients with multiple sclerosis (MS), and reviews treatment options.

TREMOR

Tremor is an involuntary rhythmic oscillation of a body part caused by alternate or synchronous contraction of agonist and antagonist muscles.[3] Rest tremor is the term given to tremors that occur when the body part is completely at rest. Action tremors

[a] Department of Neurology, University of Washington, Seattle, WA, USA; [b] Department of Neurology, Seattle VA Medical Center, University of Washington, Mailstop 127, 1660 South Columbian Way, Seattle, WA 98108, USA
* Corresponding author.
E-mail address: asamii@u.washington.edu

Phys Med Rehabil Clin N Am 24 (2013) 639–651
http://dx.doi.org/10.1016/j.pmr.2013.06.003
1047-9651/13/$ – see front matter © 2013 Elsevier Inc. All rights reserved.

can be of 3 different types: they can occur in posture when the limb is held against gravity; they can occur during movement, as in kinetic tremors; and they can present at the end of a target-guided movement, as in intention tremors.

Tremor is a common problem in MS and was in fact noted in the original triad of symptoms attributed to MS by the French neurologist Charcot,[4] the other 2 symptoms being scanning speech and nystagmus. Tremor can be seen in anywhere between 25% to 58% of patients with MS,[5,6] and has been associated with significant impairment of function and disability. Tremor is also often seen in secondary progressive MS. Estimates of the incidence of severe tremor in MS have ranged from 3% to 15%, and patients with MS tremor of any severity are more likely to be unemployed or retired early owing to disability.[5,6] Tremor in MS is most often a combination of postural and intention tremor, with the distal limb being more often involved than the proximal structures.[5] MS tremor can be bilateral and most often affects the upper limbs, although it may also involve the head, neck, or vocal cords.[7]

The pathophysiology of tremor in MS is not clear, as it rarely occurs in isolation and is usually associated with other neurologic signs and symptoms. MS tremor is thought to be mediated through the cerebellum and its connections, because of the postural and intention nature of the tremor. Rest tremors are uncommon in MS. Cooling of the limbs has been shown to reduce the intensity of the MS tremor, and this is thought to be a surrogate marker of the role of the cerebellum in MS tremor.[8] Cooling reduces muscle-spindle excitability and slows down nerve conduction, and hence likely reduces input into the tremor-producing cerebellar circuitry. The fact that upper limb tremor severity correlates highly with the degree of ataxia, dysdiadochokinesia, and dysmetria also supports the role of the cerebellar connections in the pathogenesis of MS tremor.[5] One study showed that the tremor amplitude correlated with the MS lesion load in the contralateral pons and that bilateral tremors were associated with higher lesion load in the bilateral pons, suggesting involvement of the cerebellar input and outflow pathways.[9]

Treatment of tremors in MS is challenging, which is partly due to poor response to medications but also to the associated neurologic symptoms that compound the disability. It is also difficult to segregate MS-related disability from tremor-related disability.[10] Nonpharmacologic methods used in essential tremors, such as weighted utensils and cutlery, are an option in aiding activities of daily living. Cooling the limb before activities involving precision movements such as signing documents or applying makeup has been proposed as an alternative option.[8]

Medications used for MS tremors include isoniazid, which has been shown in 2 randomized controlled trials to improve both the postural and intention components of the MS tremor. However, relatively high doses up to 1200 mg/d were needed, and this was associated with multiple side effects such as drowsiness, elevated liver function tests, and anorexia.[11,12] Animal studies have suggested a role for cannabis in improving tremor in experimental models of allergic autoimmune encephalomyelitis. However, a randomized controlled trial did not demonstrate any significant benefit.[13] In a case report, 4-aminopyridine was found to be useful in MS tremor, possibly because of its effects in improving the excitability and precision of cerebellar Purkinje cells.[14]

Topiramate has also been used successfully at low doses of 50 mg/d to control MS tremor and improve function.[15] A randomized, double-blind, placebo-controlled trial of botulinum toxin was found to reduce the severity of MS-related tremor and tremor-related disability, although a mild to moderate degree of weakness was noted in patients receiving botulinum toxin.[10] Although case series and crossover studies showed a possible role for levetiracetam in MS tremor, a randomized double-blind study failed to show any significant benefits.[16] Other medications tried include ondansetron, which has shown equivocal results,[17,18] and primidone, which showed some benefit in a pilot study wherein improvement was noted in the activities of daily living, Fahn Tremor rating scale, and nine-hole peg test in the treatment group.[19]

Surgical options for tremor in MS include lesional surgery and deep brain stimulation (DBS). Traditional targets have included the ventral intermediate and ventral oralis posterior nuclei of the thalamus. More recently, other targets such as the zona incerta and subthalamic nucleus have also been studied.[20] A systematic review of DBS in MS tremor showed improvement in tremors in up to 87% of patients, although the benefits did not appear to persist over time and reprogramming was needed.[21] Improvement in quality of life has been harder to demonstrate because of difficulties in distinguishing between MS-related disability and tremor-related disability. On rare occasions, permanent tremor reduction has been noted after DBS.[22] Such reduction can occur in the setting of weakness or independent of weakness, suggesting that this is either the natural progression of MS or a possible demyelinating "lesion effect" from long-term stimulation. One review concluded that thalamic stimulation with DBS and thalamotomy were comparable in terms of the level of tremor control, with initial tremor suppression in 93.8% of patients undergoing thalamotomy and 96% in patients undergoing DBS.[23] Functional improvement was noted more often in the thalamic stimulation group than in the thalamotomy group, and complications such as swallowing difficulties, dysarthria, hemiparesis, and balance problems were noted in both procedures.

DYSTONIAS

Dystonia is an abnormal sustained muscle contraction causing twisting or turning around 1 or multiple joints.[1] Paroxysmal dystonia, also referred to as tonic spasms, is the most frequently reported type of dystonia in MS.[24–26] This condition consists of involuntary muscle contractions of a limb or unilateral limbs that cause painful, stereotyped posturing or movements.[27] It differs from other types of dystonia in that the movements are not sustained. Instead, attacks are brief (seconds to a few minutes) and occur several times a day.[25] The proposed pathophysiologic explanation is ephaptic activation of axons secondary to a demyelinating lesion.[28,29] In cases where imaging correlation has been available, lesions have been found in the midbrain, posterior limb of the internal capsule, cerebral peduncle, thalamus, subthalamus, and cervical spinal cord.[27,30] Although the causative lesions theoretically could occur anywhere along the motor pathway, it is most likely that the spasms would be generated from sites where the motor fibers run very closely together.[28] Treatment options include a course of high-dose steroid therapy, carbamazepine,[31] acetazolamide,[30] and valproate.[28]

Cervical dystonia, also called spasmodic torticollis, is a focal dystonia affecting the neck muscles that leads to abnormal movements of the head and sustained and often painful postures of the head, neck, and shoulders.[32] It has been infrequently reported in MS patients.[33–36] Some investigators view cervical dystonia and MS as coincidental diseases.[26] In 2 of the more recent case reports, a causative relationship was thought most likely. In one case, this was based on lesions in the high cervical spine identified on magnetic resonance imaging (MRI),[36] and in the other, on the patient's response to corticotropin.[35] A sensible course of treatment for a patient with known MS presenting with cervical dystonia would be to start with a course of high-dose steroids and then, if symptoms are still present, to treat with botulinum toxin.

Occasionally, generalized dystonia and other focal dystonias, such as writer's cramp, have been reported in MS patients.[25,26,35,37] Investigators have variously postulated that the dystonia was coincidental to or caused by the MS.[25,26]

PARKINSONISM

Parkinsonism is a term that refers to a combination of signs seen in Parkinson disease, including bradykinesia, tremor, rigidity, and postural instability.[1] Although parkinsonism occurs rarely in patients with MS, there are several case reports of this phenomenon.[26,38,39] However, investigators are divided as to whether the diseases are coincidental[26,40] or whether MS lesions actually cause the parkinsonism.[38,39] It is likely that both scenarios occur. Clinical evidence in favor of a causative relationship includes the presence of MRI lesions in the midbrain or basal ganglia, and improvement with use of steroids.[38,39] Coincidental cases tend to lack such features, and patients tend to improve with levodopa therapy.[40–42]

RESTLESS LIMBS SYNDROME

Restless limbs syndrome (RLS) is a distressing desire to move the limbs, usually the legs, while sitting or lying down. Symptoms are relieved by walking. Symptoms worsen in the evening, and periodic limb movements may occur during sleep.[43] RLS is common, with a prevalence of 5% to 15%.[43] Some studies have shown a higher prevalence of RLS in MS patients,[44] whereas others did not find any association.[45] A recent large, prospective, population-based study found a significantly higher prevalence of RLS in women with MS than in women without MS: 15.5% versus 6.4%.[46] There was also a significant difference in women reporting symptoms classified as "severe RLS" when compared with women without MS: 9.9% versus 2.6%. There are different theories on the pathophysiologic link between MS and RLS. One small study showed more cervical spinal cord lesions in MS patients with RLS compared with those without RLS.[47] Iron deficiency is also associated with RLS.[48,49] Several studies have found a higher prevalence of iron deficiency anemia in MS patients than in controls, and one study noted a stronger association between RLS and MS in premenopausal than in postmenopausal women, drawing the implication that the premenopausal women likely have lower iron levels attributable to menstrual blood loss.[46] A ferritin level should be checked in RLS patients, and iron replacement considered for a ferritin level lower than 50 µg/L.[50] Identifying and treating RLS in MS patients is important because patients often have difficulty falling asleep; patients will then contend with both daytime sleepiness and the fatigue of MS. Dopamine agonists, such as ropinirole, pramipexole, and transdermal rotigotine are effective treatments for RLS.[51] Other options include carbidopa-levodopa, clonazepam, or gabapentin.

CHOREA AND BALLISMUS

Chorea, meaning "dance" in Greek, resembles exaggerated fidgetiness. The movements are usually generalized and purposeless. In mild cases, chorea may be blended into natural movements and appear purposeful.[1] Chorea has very rarely been reported in MS patients.[24,52,53] In some of these cases, the investigators deduced there was a causal association. For example, one patient with relapsing remitting MS developed widespread, bilateral chorea, and brain MRI showed bilateral involvement near the caudate nuclei.[24] Treatment options include benzodiazepines, tetrabenazine, and neuroleptic medicines such as risperidone, olanzapine, haloperidol, and fluphenazine.

Ballismus is a large-amplitude, proximal chorea, typically causing the affected limb to fling violently. It usually occurs acutely on one side of the body and is referred to as hemiballismus. It is caused most commonly by infarct in the contralateral subthalamic nucleus. There are several reported cases of hemiballismus in MS patients.[26,54–57] On

MRI, MS plaques were seen in the contralateral subthalamic nucleus in some of these patients.[56,57] Treatment options are the same as for chorea, although it would be reasonable to first try a course of steroids.[56]

MYOCLONUS

Myoclonus is a sudden, brief muscle contraction.[1] Myoclonus can localize to the cortex, subcortex, brainstem, spinal cord, and, in rare cases, the peripheral nervous system. Myoclonus is rarely reported in MS. Palatal myoclonus is the most commonly reported type.[26] Palatal myoclonus is thought to localize to lesions in the dentato-rubro-olivary pathway. In one patient with bilateral palatal myoclonus, MRI showed plaques in the pons.[58] Most MS patients with palatal myoclonus are also noted to have nystagmus.[26] Other reported cases of myoclonus in MS patients are intention myoclonus[59,60] and propriospinal myoclonus.[61] Pharmacologic treatment is the same as is recommended for myoclonus from other causes. Commonly used medications include valproic acid, clonazepam, and levetiracatem. For palatal myoclonus botulinum toxin may be effective.[62]

TICS

Tics are temporarily suppressible, abnormal movements or vocalizations.[1] The association between MS and tics is extremely rare. There has been one case report of a simple phonic tic,[63] one of a complex vocal tic,[64] and recently a report of Tourettism, which was thought to be caused by the patient's secondary progressive MS.[65] The causative link between tics and MS is difficult to make, both because of the dearth of cases that have been reported and because the precise anatomic localization of tics is not established. However, basal ganglia and the cortico-striato-thalamocortical circuit are thought to be involved,[65] and lesions were seen in those areas in the few cases reported.[63,65] Tics that are troublesome to the patient can be treated with clonidine, neuroleptic agents, benzodiazepines, or tetrabenazine.[66]

ABNORMAL FACIAL MOVEMENTS

Hemifacial spasm (HFS) is a syndrome of intermittent or sustained unilateral facial contraction that can be caused by compression of posterior fossa structures by ectatic vessels or tumors. In essential HFS there is no compressive lesion.[67] HFS is occasionally seen in MS patients.[67,68] In one case series of 6 MS patients who developed HFS, 2 of the patients had brain MRI showing lesions in the lower pons unilateral to the HFS.[67] The investigators posit that in MS patients with HFS, the lesions usually involve the facial nucleus or the proximal portion of the facial nerve. Treatment options for HFS in MS patients include corticosteroids, carbamazepine, and especially botulinum toxin.[67,69]

Spastic paretic hemifacial contracture (SPHC) is a sustained unilateral contraction of the facial muscles with ipsilateral facial paresis.[70] The condition was originally associated with brainstem tumors, but there have been a handful of case reports of SPHC in MS patients.[70,71] MRI in those cases showed pontine lesions, and symptoms resolved over a few months. SPHC is distinguishable from facial myokymia, which also occurs in MS patients, by the absence of myokymia on both examination and electromyography, and clinically there is more severe contracture in SPHC.[71]

Facial myokymia is a continuous wave-like, undulating and flickering movement affecting individual muscle fascicles.[69,72] Facial myokymia has been frequently reported in MS patients, including reports of this as the presenting sign of MS.[67,73,74]

It is thought to localize to the pontine tegmentum, specifically the postnuclear, post-genu portion of the facial nerve.[75] The most effective treatment is botulinum toxin.[74,76]

ATAXIA

Ataxia refers to impaired motor coordination that is usually related to disorders of the cerebellum or its connections with the rest of the central nervous system.[1] Ataxia is a common movement disorder found in demyelinating disease, and can cause significant disability. It is characterized by dysfunction in coordination that can involve the limbs, trunk, and/or speech. Findings in ataxia include dysmetria, whereby there is impaired generation, guidance, and termination of the movement of a limb, causing overshoot or past-pointing. Ataxia can include abnormal postural reactions, causing rebound of a limb, and dysdiadochokinesis, whereby there is an inability to perform rhythmic repetitive movements such as rapid alternating hand movements. Ataxic speech is characterized by clumsy dysarthria that has altered rate, prosody, and modulation of speech. Coordination of eye movements is also often affected, resulting in nystagmus and hypometric or hypermetric saccades. An ataxic gait is wide-based and unstable, usually requiring slower and shorter strides. Ataxia can often be associated with kinetic and postural tremor.

Ataxia is usually localized to lesions or disorders involving the cerebellum or cerebellar projections to the brain, brainstem, thalamus, and spinal cord.[77] Correlation of clinical symptoms to precise cerebellar anatomy has been difficult, but the most clinically useful anatomic divisions of the cerebellum are the midline, hemispheres, and posterior regions.[78–80] The midline of the cerebellum, which includes the vermis, is associated with truncal ataxia, titubation, and gait ataxia. Unilateral limb ataxia is usually due to lesions in the ipsilateral cerebellar hemisphere. Lesions in the posterior cerebellum, which includes the flocculonodular lobe, can cause gait ataxia and balance problems as well as eye-movement dyscoordination such as nystagmus. Cerebellar tremor is often due to lesions that extend beyond the cerebellar cortex, involving the cerebello-rubro-thalamocortical tract.[9,80] However, ataxia also has a significant component of sensory integration in coordinating movement, and a sensory ataxia can result from demyelinating lesions involving central or peripheral sensory tracts and the vestibular system.

Episodic ataxia has been reported in several patients in the context of demyelinating disease. Marcel and colleagues[81] reported two patients presenting with gait ataxia and dysarthria as initial symptoms of demyelinating disease. Both patients had midbrain lesions at the level of the red nucleus, among other subcortical white-matter lesions. The first patient initially developed subacute gait ataxia and dysarthria following a mild upper respiratory infection. The ataxia resolved with high-dose intravenous steroid treatment, but the patient subsequently developed stereotyped episodes of gait ataxia, dysmetria, and dysarthria lasting 5 to 15 seconds and occurring up to 100 times per day. The patient had multiple nonenhancing T2-hyperintense lesions in the midbrain, including 1 at the level of the red nucleus, as well as in the periventricular and subcortical white matter. The episodes of ataxia remitted with another round of intravenous steroids and oral carbamazepine. This patient did not have further evidence of demyelinating disease in space and time, and was diagnosed with a clinically isolated syndrome. The second patient presented with similar episodes of paroxysmal dysarthria-ataxia as the initial presentation for MS. Again, his symptoms lasted 5 to 15 seconds, occurring up to 150 times per day, with a normal neurologic examination between episodes. This patient was also found to have several nonenhancing T2-hyperintense lesions in the periventricular white matter and midbrain at the level of the red nucleus, as well as in the pons, cerebellum, and cervical spinal cord. The paroxysmal ataxia and dysarthria resolved with oxcarbamazepine. Li and colleagues[82] reported similar brief episodes of ataxia in two patients with demyelinating disease involving the red nucleus. Ataxic dysarthria was the presenting symptom in one of the patients, following an upper respiratory infection. Paroxysmal ataxia and dysarthria developed in the second patient after already being diagnosed with MS of 6 months' duration. The episodes resolved with carbamazepine in both patients.

Karmon and colleagues[83] reported 5 cases of limb ataxia associated with pericentral sulcus demyelinating lesions in MS. Three of the patients presented with limb ataxia as their first symptom of MS. All 5 patients had cortical and subcortical T2-FLAIR (fluid-attenuated inversion recovery) hyperintense lesions in the pericentral gyrus region contralateral to the limb ataxia without brainstem or cerebellar abnormality on MRI. Longitudinal follow-up of these patients ranging from 1.5 to 18 years revealed continued disability caused by the ataxic tremor, with 3 of the 5 patients with mild tremor, 1 with moderate tremor, and 1 with severe tremor. The patients had only partial improvement or no benefit from treatment with propranolol, benzodiazepines, levodopa, or primidone. Ataxic hemiparesis consistent with a lacunar syndrome has also been reported as a presenting symptom of MS, correlating with a hyperintense T2 lesion involving the thalamus and internal capsule contralateral to the limb ataxia.[84] These cases underscore the variety of anatomic locations where demyelinating lesions can cause ataxia, beyond the previously well-recognized cerebellar projections to the basal ganglia and brainstem. These cases also illustrate the significant long-term disability that ataxia can cause in MS patients.

Symptomatic treatment of cerebellar ataxia remains challenging. Treatment is supportive and is often multidisciplinary. Benzodiazepines and barbiturates such as clonazepam and primidone, respectively, may initially improve tremor but can cause long-term worsening of balance and coordination. Baclofen has also been reported to worsen ataxia, whereas acetazolamide and calcium-channel blockers can be effective in episodic ataxias.[78] Physical, occupational, and speech therapies, as well as rehabilitation, are important for maintaining safe ambulation and swallowing, and as much independence as possible with activities of daily living.

A systematic review of treatments for ataxia in MS identified 10 randomized controlled trials, none of which provided evidence for an effective long-term therapy for cerebellar tremor or ataxia.[85] The included studies investigated isoniazid and pyridoxine, cannabis-based medications, baclofen, thalamotomy versus DBS, and physiotherapy and neurorehabilitation. Outcomes were complicated by various measurements of tremor, including videotaped tremor examination, accelerometry, surface electromyography, self-rating scales, balance time, and stance on a force plate. Identification of a significant improvement in ataxia outcomes was also limited by small sample size.

Ten patients with MS were included in a single, blinded, randomized controlled trial for treatment of medication-resistant tremor with thalamotomy and thalamic DBS.[86] Both interventions initially improved tremor in all MS patients; however, the tremor returned in nearly all of the patients by 6 months after surgery and there was no improvement in disability scores at 6-month follow-up. There were also adverse effects in both thalamotomy and DBS treatment groups on gait, dysarthria, and arm ataxia.

Three randomized physiotherapy studies show modest improvement in function in MS patients with ataxia, although long-term benefits remain unclear. In a study of 26 secondary or primary progressive MS patients with significant ataxia randomized to physiotherapy with and without use of Johnstone pressure splints, both treatment arms had small improvement in limb stance time and step width following physiotherapy, and improvement in Expanded Disability Status Scale (EDSS) score of 0.5.[87] There was no evidence for benefit from the use of Johnstone pressure splints. A study randomizing 23 patients to two different physiotherapy approaches found small improvement in Rivermead mobility index in both treatment arms.[88] A third study randomized 42 patients with gait abnormalities to home, outpatient, or no therapy.[89] Both the home and outpatient groups had improvement in Rivermead mobility index when compared with the group with no therapy. However, follow-up 2 months after treatment found that mobility had regressed to pretreatment levels. A case report of an MS patient with severe truncal ataxia describes torso-weighting as providing long-term benefit.[90]

Topiramate was described in a case report to have long-term effectiveness on cerebellar tremor and ataxia.[15] The reported patient had a 17-year history of well-controlled relapsing-remitting MS treated with natalizumab, with significant ataxia involving the trunk, limbs, eye movements, and speech, and severe postural and kinetic cerebellar tremor. She was unable to walk more than 50 ft (15 m) with bilateral support, or dress, bathe, or eat independently because of the severity of the tremor and ataxia. Her EDSS score was 6.5. MRI revealed a high lesion load with multiple white-matter lesions involving the pons, middle cerebellar peduncles, and cerebellar hemispheres. She responded to topiramate in a sustained, dose-dependent manner, titrated up to 150 mg/d. After 2 years of topiramate treatment, she had significant functional improvement and was able to eat, drink, and dress independently, and walk 600 ft (180 m) with a walking frame. Withdrawal of topiramate led to worsening of ataxia and tremor, which improved after restarting the medication.

Levetiracetam was found to improve cerebellar tremor in a small open-label pilot tolerability and efficacy study of 14 MS patients.[91] Significant improvement was found on videotaped tremor and ataxia examination and the subjective Activities of Daily Life questionnaire after titration of levetiracetam. The medication was well tolerated, with 3 subjects withdrawing because of side effects of sedation or agitation. However, there have not yet been any further controlled, randomized studies looking at the efficacy of levetiracetam on ataxia in a larger number of MS patients.

In summary, ataxia is a common movement disorder in MS that can lead to significant disability. It is typically localized to lesions involving the cerebellum and cerebello-rubro-thalamocortical tract. However, reports have demonstrated that ataxia can be associated with lesions not involving the ipsilateral posterior fossa, such as the contralateral pericentral gyrus cortical and subcortical regions. Several case reports have highlighted a rare syndrome of brief episodic ataxia and dysarthria that can be found in the setting of demyelinating disease that is responsive to carbamazepine. Unfortunately, most ataxia is difficult to treat, and requires a multidisciplinary approach of physiotherapy, rehabilitation, and careful consideration of medications so as not to worsen it.

REFERENCES

1. Samii A, Ransom BR. Movement disorders: overview and treatment options. P&T 2005;30(4):228–41.
2. Fahn S. Classification of movement disorders. Mov Disord 2011;26(6):947–57.
3. Puschmann A, Wszolek ZK. Diagnosis and treatment of common forms of tremor. Semin Neurol 2011;31(1):65–77.
4. Shneyder N, Harris MK, Minagar A. Movement disorders in patients with multiple sclerosis. Handb Clin Neurol 2011;100:307–14.

5. Alusi SH, Worthington J, Glickman S, et al. A study of tremor in multiple sclerosis. Brain 2001;124(Pt 4):720–30.
6. Pittock SJ, McClelland RL, Mayr WT, et al. Prevalence of tremor in multiple sclerosis and associated disability in the Olmsted County population. Mov Disord 2004;19(12):1482–5.
7. Koch M, Mostert J, Heersema D, et al. Tremor in multiple sclerosis. J Neurol 2007;254(2):133–45.
8. Feys P, Helsen W, Liu X, et al. Effects of peripheral cooling on intention tremor in multiple sclerosis. J Neurol Neurosurg Psychiatry 2005;76(3):373–9.
9. Feys P, Maes F, Nuttin B, et al. Relationship between multiple sclerosis intention tremor severity and lesion load in the brainstem. Neuroreport 2005;16(12): 1379–82.
10. Van Der Walt A, Sung S, Spelman T, et al. A double-blind, randomized, controlled study of botulinum toxin type A in MS-related tremor. Neurology 2012;79(1):92–9.
11. Hallett M, Lindsey JW, Adelstein BD, et al. Controlled trial of isoniazid therapy for severe postural cerebellar tremor in multiple sclerosis. Neurology 1985;35(9): 1374–7.
12. Bozek CB, Kastrukoff LF, Wright JM, et al. A controlled trial of isoniazid therapy for action tremor in multiple sclerosis. J Neurol 1987;234(1):36–9.
13. Fox P, Bain PG, Glickman S, et al. The effect of cannabis on tremor in patients with multiple sclerosis. Neurology 2004;62(7):1105–9.
14. Schniepp R, Jakl V, Wuehr M, et al. Treatment with 4-aminopyridine improves upper limb tremor of a patient with multiple sclerosis: a video case report. Mult Scler 2012;9(4):506–8.
15. Schroeder A, Linker RA, Lukas C, et al. Successful treatment of cerebellar ataxia and tremor in multiple sclerosis with topiramate: a case report. Clin Neuropharmacol 2010;33(6):317–8.
16. Feys P, D'hooghe MB, Nagels G, et al. The effect of levetiracetam on tremor severity and functionality in patients with multiple sclerosis. Mult Scler 2009; 15(3):371–8.
17. Rice GP, Lesaux J, Vandervoort P, et al. Ondansetron, a 5-HT3 antagonist, improves cerebellar tremor. J Neurol Neurosurg Psychiatry 1997;62(3):282–4.
18. Gbadamosi J, Buhmann C, Moench A, et al. Failure of ondansetron in treating cerebellar tremor in MS patients–an open-label pilot study. Acta Neurol Scand 2001;104(5):308–11.
19. Naderi F, Javadi SA, Motamedi M, et al. The efficacy of primidone in reducing severe cerebellar tremors in patients with multiple sclerosis. Clin Neuropharmacol 2012;35(5):224–6.
20. Hyam JA, Aziz TZ, Bain PG. Post-deep brain stimulation–gradual nonstimulation dependent decrease in strength with attenuation of multiple sclerosis tremor. J Neurol 2007;254(7):854–60.
21. Wishart HA, Roberts DW, Roth RM, et al. Chronic deep brain stimulation for the treatment of tremor in multiple sclerosis: review and case reports. J Neurol Neurosurg Psychiatry 2003;74(10):1392–7.
22. Thevathasan W, Schweder P, Joint C, et al. Permanent tremor reduction during thalamic stimulation in multiple sclerosis. J Neurol Neurosurg Psychiatry 2011; 82(4):419–22.
23. Yap L, Kouyialis A, Varma TR. Stereotactic neurosurgery for disabling tremor in multiple sclerosis: thalamotomy or deep brain stimulation? Br J Neurosurg 2007; 21(4):349–54.

24. Mao CC, Gancher ST, Herndon RM. Movement disorders in multiple sclerosis. Mov Disord 1988;3(2):109–16.

25. Coleman RJ, Quinn NP, Marsden CD. Multiple sclerosis presenting as adult onset dystonia. Mov Disord 1988;3(4):329–32.

26. Tranchant C, Bhatia KP, Marsden CD. Movement disorders in multiple sclerosis. Mov Disord 1995;10(4):418–23.

27. Fontoura P, Vale J, Guimarães J. Symptomatic paroxysmal hemidystonia due to a demyelinating subthalamic lesion. Eur J Neurol 2000;7(5):559–62.

28. Andrade C, Massano J, Guimarães J, et al. Stretching the limbs? Tonic spasms in multiple sclerosis. BMJ Case Rep 2012;2012.

29. Ostermann PO, Westerberg CE. Paroxysmal attacks in multiple sclerosis. Brain 1975;98(2):189–202.

30. Waubant E, Alizé P, Tourbah A, et al. Paroxysmal dystonia (tonic spasm) in multiple sclerosis. Neurology 2001;57(12):2320–1.

31. Espir ML, Millac P. Treatment of paroxysmal disorders in multiple sclerosis with carbamazepine (Tegretol). J Neurol Neurosurg Psychiatry 1970;33(4):528–31.

32. Jost WH, Hefter H, Stenner A, et al. Rating scales for cervical dystonia: a critical evaluation of tools for outcome assessment of botulinum toxin therapy. J Neural Transm 2013;120(3):487–96.

33. Milanov I, Georgiev D. Spasmodic torticollis and tremor due to multiple sclerosis: a case report. Funct Neurol 1995;10(6):281–5.

34. Svetel M, Sternic N, Filipovic S, et al. Spasmodic torticollis associated with multiple sclerosis: report of two cases. Mov Disord 1997;12(6):1092–4.

35. Minagar A, Sheremata WA, Weiner WJ. Transient movement disorders and multiple sclerosis. Parkinsonism Relat Disord 2002;9(2):111–3.

36. Rüegg SJ, Bühlmann M, Renaud S, et al. Cervical dystonia as first manifestation of multiple sclerosis. J Neurol 2004;251(11):1408–10.

37. Bachman DS, Laó-Vélez C, Estanol B. Letter: dystonia and choreoathetosis in multiple sclerosis. Arch Neurol 1976;33(8):590.

38. Federlein J, Postert T, Allgeier A, et al. Remitting parkinsonism as a symptom of multiple sclerosis and the associated magnetic resonance imaging findings. Mov Disord 1997;12(6):1090–1.

39. Folgar S, Gatto EM, Raina G, et al. Parkinsonism as a manifestation of multiple sclerosis. Mov Disord 2003;18(1):108–10.

40. Valkovic P, Krastev G, Mako M, et al. A unique case of coincidence of early onset Parkinson's disease and multiple sclerosis. Mov Disord 2007;22(15): 2278–81.

41. Pedemonte E, Trabucco E, Cella M, et al. Parkinsonism in multiple sclerosis patients: a casual or causal association? Parkinsonism Relat Disord 2013;19(4): 492–3.

42. Barun B, Brinar VV, Zadro I, et al. Parkinsonism and multiple sclerosis—is there association? Clin Neurol Neurosurg 2008;110(9):958–61.

43. Schapira AH. Restless legs syndrome: an update on treatment options. Drugs 2004;64(2):149–58.

44. Manconi M, Ferini-Strambi L, Filippi M, et al. Multicenter case-control study on restless legs syndrome in multiple sclerosis: the REMS study. Sleep 2008; 31(7):944–52.

45. Gómez-Choco MJ, Iranzo A, Blanco Y, et al. Prevalence of restless legs syndrome and REM sleep behavior disorder in multiple sclerosis. Mult Scler 2007;13(6):805–8.

46. Li Y, Munger KL, Batool-Anwar S, et al. Association of multiple scerosis with restless legs syndrome and other sleep disorders in women. Neurology 2012; 78(19):1500–6.

47. Manconi M, Rocca MA, Ferini-Strambi L, et al. Restless legs syndrome is a common finding in multiple sclerosis and correlates with cervical cord damage. Mult Scler 2008;14(1):86–93.

48. O'Keeffe ST, Gavin K, Lavan JN. Iron status and restless legs syndrome in the elderly. Age Ageing 1994;23(3):200–3.

49. Salas RE, Gamaldo CE, Allen RP. Update in restless legs syndrome. Curr Opin Neurol 2010;23(4):401–6.

50. Ryan M, Slevin JT. Restless legs syndrome. Am J Health Syst Pharm 2006; 63(17):1599–612.

51. Leschziner G, Gringras P. Restless legs syndrome. BMJ 2012;344:e3056.

52. Sarkari NB. Involuntary movements in multiple sclerosis. Br Med J 1968;2(5607): 738–40.

53. Taff I, Sabato UC, Lehrer G. Choreoathetosis in multiple sclerosis. Clin Neurol Neurosurg 1985;87(1):41–3.

54. Mouren P, Tatossian A, Toga M, et al. Critical study of the hemiballic syndrome. (Apropos of an anatomo-clinical case of multiple sclerosis with terminal monoballistic hyperkinesia). Encephale 1966;55(3):212–74 [in French].

55. Giroud M, Semama D, Pradeaux L, et al. Hemiballismus revealing multiple sclerosis in an infant. Childs Nerv Syst 1990;6(4):236–8.

56. Waubant E, Simonetta-Moreau M, Clanet M, et al. Left arm monoballism as a relapse in multiple sclerosis. Mov Disord 1997;12(6):1091–2.

57. Riley D, Lang AE. Hemiballism in multiple sclerosis. Mov Disord 1988;3(1): 88–94.

58. Revol A, Vighetto A, Confavreux C, et al. Oculo-palatal myoclonus and multiple sclerosis. s 1990;146(8–9):518–21 [in French].

59. Hassler R, Bronisch F, Mundinger F, et al. Intention myoclonus of multiple sclerosis, its patho-anatomical basis and its stereotactic relief. Neurochirurgia (Stuttg) 1975;18(3):90–106.

60. Mukand JA, Giunti EJ. Tizanidine for the treatment of intention myoclonus: a case series. Arch Phys Med Rehabil 2004;85(7):1125–7.

61. Kapoor R, Brown P, Thompson PD, et al. Propriospinal myoclonus in multiple sclerosis. J Neurol Neurosurg Psychiatry 1992;55(11):1086–8.

62. Penney SE, Bruce IA, Saeed SR. Botulinum toxin is effective and safe for palatal tremor: a report of five cases and a review of the literature. J Neurol 2006;253(7): 857–60.

63. Lana-Peixoto MA, Teixeira AL. Brazilian Committee for Treatment and Research in Multiple Sclerosis. Simple phonic tic in multiple sclerosis. Mult Scler 2002; 8(6):510.

64. Deutsch SI, Rosse RB, Connor JM, et al. Current status of cannabis treatment of multiple sclerosis with an illustrative case presentation of a patient with MS, complex vocal tics, paroxysmal dystonia, and marijuana dependence treated with dronabinol. CNS Spectr 2008;13(5):393–403.

65. Nociti V, Fasano A, Bentivoglio AR, et al. Tourettism in multiple sclerosis: a case report. J Neurol Sci 2009;287(1–2):288–90.

66. Shprecher D, Kurlan R. The management of tics. Mov Disord 2009;24(1):15–24.

67. Telischi FF, Grobman LR, Sheremata WA, et al. Hemifacial spasm. Occurrence in multiple sclerosis. Arch Otolaryngol Head Neck Surg 1991;117(5):554–6.

68. Nociti V, Bentivoglio AR, Frisullo G, et al. Movement disorders in multiple sclerosis: causal or coincidental association? Mult Scler 2008;14(9):1284–7.

69. Wang A, Jankovic J. Hemifacial spasm: clinical findings and treatment. Muscle Nerve 1998;21(12):1740–7.

70. Koutsis G, Kokotis P, Sarrigiannis P, et al. Spastic paretic hemifacial contracture in multiple sclerosis: a neglected clinical and EMG entity. Mult Scler 2008;14(7): 927–32.

71. Sarrigiannis P, Tsakanicas C, Anagnostouli M, et al. Spastic paretic hemifacial contracture (SPHC) in a patient with multiple sclerosis. A clinical, EMG and neuroimaging study. Neurophysiol Clin 2004;34(3–4):147–51.

72. Horowitz SH. Hemifacial spasm and facial myokymia: electrophysiological findings. Muscle Nerve 1987;10(5):422–7.

73. Dupeyron A, Chaury F, Guiraud-Chaumeil C, et al. Hemicontracture and facial myokymia as the first manifestation of multiple sclerosis. Rev Neurol (Paris) 2001;157(3):315–7 [in French].

74. Habek M, Adamec I, Gabelić T, et al. Treatment of facial myokymia in multiple sclerosis with botulinum toxin. Acta Neurol Belg 2012;112(4):423–4.

75. Jacobs L, Kaba S, Pullicino P. The lesion causing continuous facial myokymia in multiple sclerosis. Arch Neurol 1994;51(11):1115–9.

76. Sedano MJ, Trejo JM, Macarrón JL, et al. Continuous facial myokymia in multiple sclerosis: treatment with botulinum toxin. Eur Neurol 2000;43(3):137–40.

77. Klockgether T, Paulson H. Milestones in ataxia. Mov Disord 2011;26(6):1134–41.

78. Perlman SL. Cerebellar ataxia. Curr Treat Options Neurol 2000;2(3):215–24.

79. Seidel K, Siswanto S, Brunt ER, et al. Brain pathology of spinocerebellar ataxias. Acta Neuropathol 2012;124(1):1–21.

80. Grimaldi G, Manto M. Topography of cerebellar deficits in humans. Cerebellum 2012;11(2):336–51.

81. Marcel C, Anheim M, Flamand-Rouvière C, et al. Symptomatic paroxysmal dysarthria-ataxia in demyelinating diseases. J Neurol 2010;257(8):1369–72.

82. Li Y, Zeng C, Luo T. Paroxysmal dysarthria and ataxia in multiple sclerosis and corresponding magnetic resonance imaging findings. J Neurol 2011;258(2): 273–6.

83. Karmon Y, Morrow SA, Weinstock A, et al. Limb ataxia originating from pericentral sulcus demyelinating lesion in multiple sclerosis. J Neurol Sci 2012; 320(1–2):136–40.

84. Gorman MJ. Multiple sclerosis presenting as ataxic hemiparesis. J Neurol Sci 2002;197(1–2):85–7.

85. Mills RJ, Yap L, Young CA. Treatment for ataxia in multiple sclerosis. Cochrane Database Syst Rev 2007;(1):CD005029.

86. Schuurman PR, Bosch DA, Bossuyt PM, et al. A comparison of continuous thalamic stimulation and thalamotomy for suppression of severe tremor. N Engl J Med 2000;342(7):461–8.

87. Armutlu K, Karabudak R, Nurlu G. Physiotherapy approaches in the treatment of ataxic multiple sclerosis: a pilot study. Neurorehabil Neural Repair 2001;15(3): 203–11.

88. Lord SE, Wade DT, Halligan PW. A comparison of two physiotherapy treatment approaches to improve walking in multiple sclerosis: a pilot randomized controlled study. Clin Rehabil 1998;12(6):477–86.

89. Wiles CM, Newcombe RG, Fuller KJ, et al. Controlled randomised crossover trial of the effects of physiotherapy on mobility in chronic multiple sclerosis. J Neurol Neurosurg Psychiatry 2001;70(2):174–9.

90. Gibson-Horn C. Balance-based torso-weighting in a patient with ataxia and multiple sclerosis: a case report. J Neurol Phys Ther 2008;32(3):139–46.
91. Striano P, Coppola A, Vacca G, et al. Levetiracetam for cerebellar tremor in multiple sclerosis: an open-label pilot tolerability and efficacy study. J Neurol 2006; 253(6):762–6.

Multiple Sclerosis and Fatigue
Understanding the Patient's Needs

Karon F. Cook, PhD[a],*, Alyssa M. Bamer, MPH[b],
Toni S. Roddey, PT, PhD[c], George H. Kraft, MD, MS[d,e],
Jiseon Kim, PhD[b], Dagmar Amtmann, PhD[b]

KEYWORDS

- Multiple sclerosis • Fatigue • Outcomes assessment • Psychometrics

KEY POINTS

- Fatigue substantially affects the quality of life of persons with multiple sclerosis (MS).
- A sample of individuals living with MS ranked a subset of self-report items with respect to their relevance in measuring fatigue in MS. The most highly ranked items were, "How often did you feel tired even when you haven't done anything," and "How often did you have to push yourself to get things done because of your fatigue?"
- No self-report measure can gather the detailed and personally relevant information that can be elicited by a skilled clinician. It is possible, however, that standardized measures may pave the way for such communication.

INTRODUCTION

Fatigue is among the most common and debilitating symptoms of multiple sclerosis (MS), affecting approximately 80% of persons who have the disease.[1–4] In one study,

Disclosures: Dr G. Kraft is a member of the Medical advisory board for ACCORDA, the Advisory Board of NCMRR, and the Advisory Board of the Kessler Research Institute at UMDNJ.
Funding Sources: The contents of this article were developed under a grant from the Department of Education, NIDRR grant number H133B080025. However, those contents do not necessarily represent the policy of the Department of Education, and endorsement by the Federal Government should not be assumed. Dr Cook: NIDRR, NIH, AHRQ; Dr Bamer: NIDRR; Dr Kraft: NIDRR; Dr Kim: NIDRR; Dr Amtmann: NIH, NIDRR, CMSC.
[a] Department of Medical Social Sciences, Northwestern University Feinberg School of Medicine, 625 North Michigan Avenue, Suite 2700, Chicago, IL 60611, USA; [b] Department of Rehabilitation Medicine, School of Medicine, University of Washington, Box 354237, Seattle, WA 98195-4237, USA; [c] School of Physical Therapy, College of Health Sciences, Texas Woman's University, 6700 Fannin Street, Houston, TX 77030, USA; [d] Department of Rehabilitation Medicine, MSRRTC, University of Washington, 1959 Northeast Pacific Street, Box 356490, Seattle, WA 98195-6490, USA; [e] Department of Neurology, MSRRTC, University of Washington, 1959 Northeast Pacific Street, Box 356490, Seattle, WA 98195-6490, USA
* Corresponding author. Department of Medical Social Sciences, Northwestern University Feinberg School of Medicine, 625 North Michigan Avenue, Suite 2700, Chicago, IL 60611.
E-mail address: karon.cook@northwestern.edu

Phys Med Rehabil Clin N Am 24 (2013) 653–661
http://dx.doi.org/10.1016/j.pmr.2013.06.006
1047-9651/13/$ – see front matter © 2013 Elsevier Inc. All rights reserved.

69% considered fatigue their worst symptom.[5] Fatigue in MS may directly affect participation in important roles such as employment,[6,7] and can profoundly magnify other MS symptoms.[8]

Because fatigue is a subjective experience for which currently there is no laboratory measurement test, the assessment of fatigue typically is accomplished through self-report. In recent years standardized self-report measures have been developed using an item-banking approach.[9] Recently, as part of the National Institutes of Health Patient Reported Outcome Measurement Information System (PROMIS), a bank of items was developed for measuring self-reported fatigue.[10] In the PROMIS domain framework fatigue is defined as "an overwhelming, debilitating, and sustained sense of exhaustion that decreases one's ability to carry out daily activities, including the ability to work effectively and to function at one's usual level in family or social roles."[11(p1318)]

This study described herein had two purposes. The first was to assess, from the perspective of individuals living with MS, the relevance of a subset of items from the PROMIS fatigue item bank. The second was to identify additional aspects of fatigue that individuals with MS believed were important for clinicians when asking about their fatigue experience.

METHODS
Participants

Approval was obtained from the institutional review board of the appropriate institutions for the study, and all rights of human subjects were protected in this research. Participants were recruited through a Web site and print advertisements as well as from a disability registry maintained at the University of Washington, Seattle (UW). Individuals in the registry who had MS were sent an invitation letter followed by a phone call to assess their interest in participation.

Procedures

To evaluate the level of fatigue in the sample, the survey began with the item, "To what degree have you experienced fatigue?"[12] The item was scored on a numerical rating scale of 0 to 10, where 0 = "not at all" and 10 = "a great deal".

Item rankings

A sorting and ranking procedure was designed to quantify, from the perspective of persons with MS, the relevance of items in the PROMIS fatigue bank. The full item bank consists of 95 items, which was judged to be too many for individuals to meaningfully rank. Study investigators reduced the items to 20 in a series of successive steps described in detail elsewhere.[13] To summarize, the item pool was reduced to 44 items by eliminating items with duplicate content. These 44 items were ranked by 27 physical therapists, 7 medical doctors, and 3 occupational therapists. Based on their ratings and on cumulative coverage of content, the item pool was further reduced to the 20 items ultimately presented to participants.

The selected items were printed onto 20 2 × 3.5-inch paper note cards and mailed to participants along with written instructions for the ranking procedure. Participants first responded to the question, "To what degree have you experienced fatigue?" Responses ranged from 0 (not at all) to 10 (a great deal). Next, participants identified and recorded the 3 items of the 20 that they considered the most relevant to their fatigue. Instructions stated: "If your doctor were to ask you 3 (only 3) questions about your fatigue, what 3 questions would give your doctor the best description of your fatigue?" Next, participants selected the item from those remaining that they would want to be asked if they could add just one more question. This procedure was repeated until participants had chosen a total of 10 items. The 3 items selected as giving "the best description" were assigned a ranking of 8. The fourth item selected was assigned a ranking of 7, and so on through the tenth item that was assigned a ranking of 1. Thus, higher values indicated stronger preference.

Open-ended responses
After identifying and ranking their top 10 items, participants were asked, "Are there other questions (ones not printed on the cards) that you think are needed for a good summary of your fatigue?" Space was provided for participants to write responses.

Analysis

Item rankings
The item rankings provided by participants were ordinal-level, not interval-level, data; therefore, the appropriate average of these ranks is the median. However, because only 10 items per person received a rank (all others were scored as 0), the median rankings for most items was 0. To better discriminate among item ranks, the arithmetical mean rank across raters was calculated, which is referred to hereafter as the relevance index (RI). The authors note that this index provides relative (not equal-interval level) information about the strength of participant preferences for one item over another.

Open-ended responses
Responses to the open-ended questions were categorized according to recurring themes. Two of the study investigators (K.F.C. and A.M.B.) independently reviewed participant responses and developed categories that they thought adequately summarized the content of responses. The investigators then met and came to agreement on names and number of organizing categories. Each investigator again reviewed responses and categorized them into the agreed-upon categories. After making classifications independently, they met and compared results, resolving discrepancies by consensus.

RESULTS
Participants

Of 31 invited individuals with MS from the UW registry, 21 (68%) agreed to participate and completed the sorting procedure. Forty-one additional subjects saw a study advertisement or heard about the study from someone else and contacted the researchers directly. Of these 41, 25 (61%) subsequently completed the sorting procedure, for a grand total of 46 participants with MS. Characteristics of the participants are reported in **Table 1**.

Item Rankings

RI values were calculated for each of the 20 items reviewed by participants and are listed in **Table 2**. As the table reports, the 2 items with the highest rankings were, "How often did you feel tired even when you hadn't done anything?" and "How often did you have to push yourself to get things done because of your fatigue?" Other highly ranked items had to do with feeling tired and fatigue's impact on "finishing things," "physical function," and "thinking clearly."

Four of the 6 lowest ranked items were related to participation (ie, socializing with family, recreational activities, leaving the house, and participating in social activities). The other 2 low-ranked items asked about the impact of fatigue on bathing/showering and about frequency of experiencing "extreme exhaustion."

Table 1 Participant demographics and fatigue ratings of 0 to 10	
Demographics	
Age (y)	Mean = 54.1, SD = 9.3
Disease duration (y)	Mean = 14.1, SD = 8.2
Female	n = 37 (80.4%)
Fatigue (0–10 scale)	
None (0)	n = 2 (4.3%)
Mild (1)	n = 0 (0%)
Moderate (2–4)	n = 5 (10.8%)
Severe (5–10)	n = 39 (84.8%)

Abbreviation: SD, standard deviation.

Open-Ended Responses

Of the 46 participants, 30 made a total of 68 item suggestions in response to the query, "What other information should be asked in addition to the top ten questions you selected?" After reviewing the content of open-ended responses, study investigators identified 7 recurring themes and 2 comments that each formed its own category. One of these was the suggestion to ask "questions relating to sexual relations." Another recommended that the opportunity be given "to comment with greater detail." The complete results are reported in **Table 3**. Many of the participant suggestions were consistent with content typically represented in standardized fatigue measures. Of the 68 suggestions, 13 pertained to impact of fatigue on activities of daily living (ADLs) and instrument ADLs (IADLs), 5 pertained to cognitive impact, and 10 had concerned the emotional impact of fatigue.

A substantial number of suggestions, however, referenced content not typically covered in standardized fatigue measures. Twelve comments pertained to fatigue triggers (eg, "How does the heat affect your fatigue?"). Eleven suggested adding questions that had to do with duration, frequency, or other temporal aspects of fatigue (eg, "What time of day are you most fatigued?"). Ten comments pertained to the specifics of how individuals coped with their fatigue (eg, "How often do you plan a nap into your day in order to have the energy to do an activity later in the day?"). Another area of concern for participants was the distinction between their fatigue and other symptoms and functions (ie, pain, physical function, bladder, vision, depression). For example, one participant suggested the item, "Do you feel you can't get out of the house due to physical fatigue or is it due to the depressive elements of the disease?"

DISCUSSION

This study documented the relevance of a subset of items of the PROMIS Fatigue item bank in a convenience sample of individuals with MS, and identified the items participants believed had the greatest relevance to their experience of fatigue. In previous work, the authors used these rankings and similar rankings by clinicians to develop the PROMIS FatigueMS, an 8-item short form derived from the PROMIS fatigue item bank.[13] However, it was clear from the input of persons with MS that the content covered by this subset of items did not exhaust what they believed clinicians should ask them in trying to understand their fatigue. When asked to suggest additional items that would give their health care provider the "best description" of their fatigue,

Table 2
Relevance index values (mean participant ranking) for items from the Patient Reported Outcomes Information System (PROMIS) fatigue item bank

PROMIS Item Name	Item Content	Relevance Index
FATEXP6	How often did you feel tired even when you hadn't done anything?	4.39
FATIMP3	How often did you have to push yourself to get things done because of your fatigue?	4.37
FATIMP16	How often did you have trouble finishing things because of your fatigue?	3.82
FATIMP49	To what degree did your fatigue interfere with your physical functioning?	3.67
FATEXP48	How often did you find yourself getting tired easily?	3.37
FATIMP30	How often were you too tired to think clearly?	3.26
FATIMP33	How often did your fatigue limit you at work (include work at home)?	3.17
FATEXP7	How often did you feel your fatigue was beyond your control?	2.76
FATIMP14	How often did your fatigue make it difficult to organize your thoughts when doing things at work (include work at home)?	2.63
FATEXP26	How often were you too tired to enjoy life?	2.43
FATIMP17	How often did your fatigue make it difficult to make decisions?	2.13
FATEXP34	How tired did you feel on average?	2.09
FATIMP9	How often did you fatigue make it difficult to plan activities ahead of time?	2.09
FATEXP21	How fatigued were you when your fatigue was at its worst?	2.07
FATIMP4	How often did your fatigue interfere with your social activities?	1.93
FATEXP5	How often did you experience extreme exhaustion?	1.93
FATIMP29	How often were you too tired to leave the house?	1.91
FATIMP21	How often were you too tired to take a bath or shower?	1.34
FATIMP15	How often did your fatigue interfere with your ability to engage in recreational activities?	1.15
FATIMP26	How often were you too tired to socialize with your family?	0.67

participants included items about coping strategies, distinguishing fatigue from other experiences, fatigue triggers, and temporal aspects of fatigue. These suggestions were consistent with the self-management challenges of living with MS and the documented impact of fatigue on quality of life.[3,4] Participants' comments demonstrated their desire to discuss such issues with the clinicians who treat them.

This finding has implications for the use of self-report measures in clinical practice. Recent studies have documented both the feasibility and the advantages of

Table 3
Participant comments classified by category

Item/Statement	Category
Because of your fatigue, do you find your personal hygiene sliding?	ADL/IADL Impact
Because of your fatigue, do you find yourself compromising (letting things slide)?	ADL/IADL Impact
Because of your fatigue, do you find yourself skipping meals or eating late or making smaller meals?	ADL/IADL Impact
Do you fall asleep while doing things you want to do like watching a good movie, being on computer or reading a book?	ADL/IADL Impact
Does fatigue affect your handwriting? Computer skills?	ADL/IADL Impact
After a shower/bath and getting dressed, do you feel you expended most of your energy?	ADL/IADL Impact
Ask questions regarding specific activities of daily living that are being affected by fatigue; dressing, meal preparation, organization within home, paying bills on time, making and keeping appointments	ADL/IADL Impact
Ask questions regarding specific activities of daily living that are being affected by fatigue; dressing, meal preparation, organization within home, paying bills on time, making and keeping appointments	ADL/IADL Impact
Did you ever get part way through a project and you were alone and thought "oh oh I bit off more than I can chew! Now what do I do?!"	ADL/IADL Impact
Does your brain or your body parts tell you "when is enough". Sometimes you try something and right away or part way your brain says oh! oh!	ADL/IADL Impact
Getting dressed, put on makeup, take care of pets, fixing something healthy for meals, especially living alone	ADL/IADL Impact
How often are you too tired to plan/cook a meal at the end of the day?	ADL/IADL Impact
How often do you get "fast food" because you are too tired to cook/plan a meal	ADL/IADL Impact
How often do you not have the energy for "unplanned" activities?	ADL/IADL Impact
Because of your fatigue, did you come to realize you made improper decisions?	Cognitive
How does using your cognitive drain you?	Cognitive
Did you feel like fatigue affected your memory?	Cognitive
Do you feel at times you are in a mental fog?	Cognitive
Do you have difficulty saying what you mean?	Cognitive
Does a nap at certain times of day help manage fatigue?	Coping
How often do stimulants help?	Coping
How often do you take "energy boosters" (stimulants, caffeinated beverages, chocolate, medication) to decrease your fatigue?	Coping
Realizing your fatigue, do you think you could have done things differently?	Coping
What do you do to stabilize situations?	Coping
How do I recover?	Coping

(continued on next page)

Table 3 (continued)	
Item/Statement	**Category**
How often do you plan a nap into your day in order to have the energy to do an activity later in the day?	Coping
Need to ask demographic questions about effect of medication on fatigue	Coping
What did you do to lessen your fatigue?	Coping
What do you do when fatigued?	Coping
At what point in a typical day do you "run out of gas?"	Temporal
How fatigued do you feel upon waking in the morning?	Temporal
How often after a busy active day are you so tired that the following day you spend resting?	Temporal
What time of day are you most fatigued?	Temporal
Does the change of seasons influence your fatigue?	Temporal
How long do bouts of fatigue last?	Temporal
How long to recover?	Temporal
Is there a time of day that you experience fatigue regularly?	Temporal
Perhaps inquiring about a person's fatigue and how it progresses (or doesn't) throughout a typical day	Temporal
What/when are your best times during a typical day?	Temporal
Do you ever feel like life is going by and think what's the point?	Emotional Impact
Does your fatigue affect your happiness?	Emotional Impact
Does your fatigue affect your overall well being and satisfaction with life?	Emotional Impact
How does it affect the quality of life for you?	Emotional Impact
How often does fatigue cause short temper?	Emotional Impact
How often does fatigue decrease patience with yourself?	Emotional Impact
How often do you just not care about people or getting things done?	Emotional Impact
How often do you reflect back to what you used to accomplish in a day?	Emotional Impact
Questions regarding fatigue and mood	Emotional Impact
Do you feel like your fatigue is a problem?	Emotional Impact
Does pain interfere with fatigue?	Symptom Interaction
How often do you think that if you could eliminate or reduce your pain you would have less fatigue?	Symptom Interaction
How often does fatigue interfere with physical function?	Symptom Interaction
Do you feel you can't get out of the house due to physical fatigue or is it due to the depressive elements of the disease?	Symptom Interaction
How fatigue effects bladder and eye sight control?	Symptom Interaction
Have you noticed any patterns/triggers for your fatigue?	Triggers
How does the heat affect your cognitive?	Triggers
How does the heat affect your fatigue?	Triggers
How often did background noise affect your fatigue?	Triggers
How often did stress affect your fatigue?	Triggers

(continued on next page)

Table 3 (continued)	
Item/Statement	Category
What fatigues you more—walking or things done with your hands and arms?	Triggers
What has changed in your life?	Triggers
Have you had any other illness in the past 7 days?	Triggers
How often did heat affect your fatigue?	Triggers
Is your fatigue triggered at certain times of day?	Triggers
What are my daily activities and which are most tiring?	Triggers
What has been going on in family life, work life, social life in the past 7 days?	Triggers
I think there needs to be an opportunity to comment with greater detail	General Comment
Questions relating to sexual relations	Impact on Sex

Abbreviations: ADL, activities of daily living; IADL, instrumental activities of daily living.

incorporating patient-reported outcome measures into clinical practice.[14,15] However, these studies do not address the need to assess concerns that cannot effectively be evaluated using standardized measures. No self-report measure can gather the detailed and personally relevant information that a skilled clinician is able to elicit. Nor can a self-report measure replace the trust built when there is effective communication between a health care provider and a patient. It is possible, however, that standardized measures may pave the way for such communication. In one randomized controlled trial, the use of self-report measures along with graphical feedback significantly increased the frequency with which health-related quality of life issues were discussed between doctors and patients in a clinical setting.[16]

This study had several limitations. The convenience sample used was relatively small (N = 46) and was taken from a single geographic area. Therefore, the results may not generalize to other individuals with MS. In addition, it is well known that there are many confounders of MS fatigue, such as depression, pain, and sleep disturbances, none of which were addressed in the current study.

SUMMARY

Future studies should evaluate the generalizability of these findings. Future efforts in measurement development should examine both the challenges of incorporating standardized assessments of fatigue into clinical practice and the role of these assessments in facilitating communication between clinical providers and individuals with MS.

REFERENCES

1. Chwastiak LA, Gibbons LE, Ehde DM, et al. Fatigue and psychiatric illness in a large community sample of persons with multiple sclerosis. J Psychosom Res 2005;59(5):291–8.
2. Kraft GH, Freal JE, Coryell JK. Disability, disease duration, and rehabilitation service needs in multiple sclerosis: patient perspectives. Arch Phys Med Rehabil 1986;67(3):164–8.

3. Amato MP, Ponziani G, Rossi F, et al. Quality of life in multiple sclerosis: the impact of depression, fatigue and disability. Mult Scler 2001;7(5):340–4.
4. Johnson SL. The concept of fatigue in multiple sclerosis. J Neurosci Nurs 2008; 40(2):72–7.
5. Fisk JD, Pontefract A, Ritvo PG, et al. The impact of fatigue on patients with multiple sclerosis. Can J Neurol Sci 1994;21(1):9–14.
6. O'Connor AB, Schwid SR, Herrmann DN, et al. Pain associated with multiple sclerosis: systematic review and proposed classification. Pain 2008;137(1):96–111.
7. Pompeii LA, Moon SD, McCrory DC. Measures of physical and cognitive function and work status among individuals with multiple sclerosis: a review of the literature. J Occup Rehabil 2005;15(1):69–84.
8. Hubsky EP, Sears JH. Fatigue in multiple sclerosis: guidelines for nursing care. Rehabil Nurs 1992;17(4):176–80.
9. Cook KF, O'Malley KJ, Roddey TS. Dynamic assessment of health outcomes: time to let the CAT out of the bag? Health Serv Res 2005;40(5 Pt 2):1694–711.
10. Lai JS, Cella D, Choi S, et al. How item banks and their applications can influence measurement practice in rehabilitation medicine: a PROMIS fatigue item bank example. Arch Phys Med Rehabil 2011;92:S20–7.
11. Riley WT, Rothrock N, Bruce B, et al. Patient-reported outcomes measurement information system (PROMIS) domain names and definitions revisions: further evaluation of content validity in IRT-derived item banks. Qual Life Res 2010; 19(9):1311–21.
12. Belza BL, Henke CJ, Yelin EH, et al. Correlates of fatigue in older adults with rheumatoid arthritis. Nurse Res 1993;42(2):93–9.
13. Cook KF, Bamer AM, Roddey TS, et al. A PROMIS fatigue short form for use by individuals who have multiple sclerosis. Qual Life Res 2012;21(6):1021–30.
14. Gurland B, Alves-Ferreira PC, Sobol T, et al. Using technology to improve data capture and integration of patient-reported outcomes into clinical care: pilot results in a busy colorectal unit. Dis Colon Rectum 2010;53(8):1168–75.
15. Gutteling JJ, Busschbach JJ, de Man RA, et al. Logistic feasibility of health related quality of life measurement in clinical practice: results of a prospective study in a large population of chronic liver patients. Health Qual Life Outcomes 2008;6:97.
16. Detmar SB, Muller MJ, Schornagel JH, et al. Health-related quality-of-life assessments and patient-physician communication: a randomized controlled trial. JAMA 2002;288(23):3027–34.

Cognition, Cognitive Dysfunction, and Cognitive Rehabilitation in Multiple Sclerosis

Mary Pepping, PhD, ABPP-CN[a],*, Julie Brunings, MS-CCC, BC-ANCDS[b], Myron Goldberg, PhD, ABPP-CN[a]

KEYWORDS

- Cognition • Cognitive rehabilitation • Cognitive retraining • Multiple sclerosis
- Cognitive dysfunction

KEY POINTS

- Nature of cognitive dysfunction in MS: complex attention, memory acquisition and retrieval, speed of information processing, and both the neurocognitive and neurobehavioral features of executive functions can all be disrupted in the context of often well-preserved basic intelligence.
- Importance of comprehensive evaluation: this should include at a minimum a thorough neuropsychological evaluation and clinical observations of the treating cognitive rehabilitation specialist.
- Pathophysiology of MS: implications for neurocognitive and neurobehavioral changes: subcortical lesions exert a clear adverse effect on complex attention, memory retrieval, and frontal-subcortical executive functions, with inflammatory and degenerative processes each playing a unique role in the background strengths and weaknesses of the individual with particular forms of MS.
- Cognitive rehabilitation: sophisticated cognitive rehabilitation approaches combine clinicians' understanding of each person's particular neurocognitive and neurobehavioral strengths and difficulties, along with training of specific strategies designed to reduce the negative functional effects of the problem areas.

INTRODUCTION

Cognitive functioning problems are common in multiple sclerosis (MS), occurring in at least half of all persons with the disorder.[1,2] Although the patterns of neuropsychological disruption in people with MS are well known (ie, attention, memory acquisition and

[a] Department of Rehabilitation Medicine, University of Washington School of Medicine, Box 356490, 1959 Northeast Pacific Street, Seattle, WA 98195, USA; [b] Rehabilitation Therapy Department, University of Washington Medical Center, Box 356154, 1959 Northeast Pacific Street, Seattle, WA 98195, USA
* Corresponding author.
E-mail address: mpepping@u.washington.edu

Phys Med Rehabil Clin N Am 24 (2013) 663–672
http://dx.doi.org/10.1016/j.pmr.2013.06.009
1047-9651/13/$ – see front matter © 2013 Elsevier Inc. All rights reserved.

retrieval, speed of information processing, and features of executive functions can be adversely affected[1–8]), much variability exists. A comprehensive neuropsychological evaluation is critical to effectively identify the set of neurologic and reactive disruptions for each person with MS.[9] The expert cognitive rehabilitation specialist also gathers pertinent formal test data and important interview information at the start of therapy to guide the plan of treatment. Observations by the treating clinician of the person's cognitive retraining needs as well as clinical data regarding effectiveness of selected strategies and approaches are key components of on-going evaluation for maximal treatment effectiveness. All of these strategies also allow the clinician to provide feedback to the person with MS about their residual strengths and the various practical applications of those strengths to support improved function and hope.

The literature on typically preserved versus disrupted neuropsychological functions in people with MS has been well established over the last 25 years or more of study.[1,2,6] The time of onset, range of affected features, and degree of severity may vary with each person's disease presentation and subtype (relapsing remitting MS, primary progressive MS, secondary progressive MS, and clinical isolated syndrome[10,11]) in the particular context of their long-standing premorbid skills and difficulties. However, for most people with MS,[1,2,4,7,8,12] the subcortical changes associated with white matter disease produce predictable problems in thinking. Lesion extension into cortical gray matter can occur,[13] as can some degree of atrophy over lengthy disease course,[14] in some individuals with MS.

As we learn more about the underlying neurophysiology of MS (eg, lesion load, gray matter involvement, atrophy, and brain regions particularly vulnerable to disruption), we are in a better position to anticipate, understand, and treat residual neurocognitive and neurobehavioral difficulties. Given what is known about the initial primarily subcortical nature of disruptions and relative sparing in most instances of cortical functions, likely strengths can also be anticipated. This knowledge of residual strengths and difficulties can give clinicians and the patient a template to develop pertinent strategies and procedures to support current function and help establish effective overlearned systems for maximal future function to the fullest extent possible.

Clinicians appreciate that these changes induced by MS do not occur in the abstract. They occur each time in a specific person who is trying to find the best way to live fully and with meaning despite the challenging constellation of symptoms caused by MS. It is the thesis of this article that the cognitive problems that result from MS can be anticipated, understood via appropriate examination, and then treated to support improved performance. We would also like the reader to expand their notion of cognitive changes to include both the neurocognitive (eg, memory retrieval problems) and neurobehavioral (eg, reduced awareness, impulsivity adversely affecting problem solving) dysfunction, which is important to address when designing treatment interventions. It is also important to appreciate premorbid personality strengths and vulnerabilities as well as reactive emotional concerns and physical symptoms that can adversely affect thinking performance. First, an overview is presented of the neuroanatomy, neuropathology, and neurophysiology relevant to MS and the particular brain structures and processes that underlie areas of disrupted versus preserved cognitive function.

PATHOPHYSIOLOGY OF MS

MS is considered to be an autoimmune-related disorder of the central nervous system, affecting initially the myelin sheath of axons. The cause of this autoimmune variant is unknown but is believed to involve an interaction of genetic and environmental factors. Brain and spinal cord regions are vulnerable. An inflammatory process at the myelin sheath site is considered to be a hallmark initial change in MS. As this process evolves, axonal damage and scarring have been shown.[15,16] Axonal damage has been associated with loss of axonal integrity and degeneration, which can give rise to cerebral atrophy.[17] MS-related disability is considered to stem from 2 processes: acute inflammatory demyelination and axonal degeneration.[18]

Although MS is often considered a disorder affecting only subcortical white matter, there is considerable evidence that cortical demyelination can also occur, even at the early stages of the disease.[13] That both subcortical and cortical brain regions can be affected in MS indicates the diffuse nature of the disease and, in turn, the risk for a widespread set of cognitive functioning problems. However, despite the potential for diffuse brain involvement, MS lesions do tend to locate in the periventricular white matter, cerebellum, and brainstem.[19,20]

Through structural neuroimaging, several MS-related pathophysiologic changes have been examined in the literature as risks for cognitive functioning difficulties.[21] Among these visualized changes, lesion load (also referred to as lesion burden), lesion location, and global or regional atrophy have received the most attention. Lesion load refers to the number of lesions identified on brain imaging within a given area and has been shown in numerous studies to be correlated positively with greater cognitive impairment.[22,23] For example, Moriarty and colleagues[24] reported a positive correlation between juxtacortical lesion load and memory dysfunction in persons with MS. Bermel and colleagues[25] noted the role of frontal lobe disease in executive dysfunction in MS.

Global atrophy and regional brain atrophy have also been found to be especially associated with cognitive dysfunction.[14,25] Neocortical volume loss has been shown to differentiate cognitively impaired and cognitively intact individuals with MS.[26] Moreover, in 2 studies by Benedict and colleagues,[26,27] the relative contribution of brain atrophy to cognitive impairment was greater than lesion burden, whereas width of the third ventricle was more highly associated with cognitive dysfunction than was whole brain atrophy.

More specifically, in some studies,[28] cognitive impairment and thalamic atrophy were linked in people with MS, particularly men.[29] The reason for the sex difference is not clear, but the central role of the thalamus as a relay station for transmission of information among and between frontal cortex, basal ganglia, and other cortical regions could explain why atrophy there would have such an important deleterious effect on key frontal-subcortical functions.

COMPREHENSIVE ASSESSMENT

In the neurorehabilitation setting, effectively evaluating and treating patients with acquired brain dysfunction requires a thorough understanding of the person's abilities, difficulties, reactions, and preferences. This understanding is essential to designing and delivering effective treatment. Although there is a role for briefer examinations in some circumstances to identify and document possible cognitive changes in MS,[30] a brief examination alone is not typically sufficient to fully elucidate the nature of the person's skills and deficits for optimal treatment planning purposes. It also does not obtain much information about personality style or features, which can augment or impede ability to participate and benefit from treatment, as natural premorbid factors or personality changes that may be developing with cortical atrophy.[31] Hence, we typically use comprehensive standardized evaluations at the start of care.

These evaluations include at a minimum in-depth neuropsychological evaluation and may include formal speech and language evaluation and occupational therapy evaluation of higher-level activities of daily living.

We would like to broaden readers' view of cognitive evaluation in MS to include the kind of on-going evaluative observation that is an integral part of the treating clinician's role as they actively modify or refine treatment strategies and advice to fit the problems observed in the person's performance. This performance can include the quality of the person's in-session work, completed homework assignments, or other functional behavior (eg, observations of relevant behavior in the waiting room). For example, is the person rifling through a large messy backpack full of papers trying to find a homework assignment despite all attempts to impose some organizational structure? Perhaps it is time to rethink the strategies or approaches being used.

A clinic-based therapist can also make note of the person's ability to keep appointments, to show up on time for those appointments, to bring with them requested materials, and to complete other scheduled activities for the week. It is easy to check if the person has important items with them every session (eg, wallet or purse, keys, phone, schedule, note-taking device or materials). Feedback in the form of test or course grades for those in college or work performance evaluations for employed people also provides objective information regarding improvements in function. Including the person's family member periodically allows the clinician to obtain observer updates on accomplishments in the home and community setting (eg, taking medications independently, better follow-through with completion of chores, improved efficiency of verbal communication, jotting down notes to aid memory performance).

COGNITIVE REHABILITATION (COGNITIVE RETRAINING)

Cognitive rehabilitation is indebted to the early pioneers of these techniques[32] in the traumatic brain injury (TBI) population and evidence-based reviews of cognitive rehabilitation efficacy[33] for people with TBI and other acquired neurologic dysfunction.

Cognitive retraining focuses on reducing cognitive impairment, developing compensatory strategies to minimize the impact of the deficits, and increasing awareness of impact of those deficits in daily activities. Impaired learning and memory (ie, efficient acquisition and retrieval) as well as slowed information processing and impaired working memory, which can adversely affect complex attention and other cognitive abilities (eg, verbal fluency, executive functions), have all been identified as primary cognitive difficulties associated with MS.[34,35]

In addition to the known disruptions that can occur in attention, memory and new learning, speed of information processing, and features of executive function,[36] people with MS have unique additional vulnerabilities. These vulnerabilities can include variability in day-to-day performance secondary to waxing and waning of MS symptoms as well as additional problems with fatigue, paresthesia, or heat sensitivity. This variability must be taken into account when designing and delivering strategies for effective cognitive retraining. Periodic review and updated modification of cognitive rehabilitation needs and strategies over time is also recommended for people with MS and their families to help maximize maintenance of adaptive functions.

Even although research evaluating cognitive retraining for MS is in its infancy, it points toward neurorehabilitation being beneficial for people with various types of cognitive problems caused by MS.[37] Research specifically related to MS supports cognitive rehabilitation of impairments in the area of executive functioning,[37] as do expert opinion articles.[38] The TBI literature shows evidence to support a practice standard of metacognitive approaches for treating deficits in planning and problem solving.[39] Both the MS and TBI literature identify training in the use of compensatory techniques for memory as a practice guideline.[37,40–42]

The TBI literature has long supported the use of cognitive rehabilitation for improved attention.[33,43] Although additional evidence is still being gathered for specific MS populations,[37] it is reasonable to consider that people with MS, for whom the ability to sustain attention on relevant targets or topics and to filter competing stimuli is a main concern of treatment, can benefit from established approaches. As further research is conducted, many of the treatment approaches in use based on clinical usefulness and observed improvements in function for people with MS seem likely to achieve practice standard or practice guideline status.

Treatment Planning Interview with Patient and Family

Developing a treatment plan for cognitive retraining must begin, as noted earlier, with effective evaluation. One of the most critical yet sometimes neglected elements of evaluation for treatment planning is a systematic interview with the patient and family member or significant other by the treating clinician at the outset of treatment. It is important to understand the functional impact of impairment in order to tailor the treatment plan and compensatory strategies to meet an individual's needs. Interview questions can probe for specific examples of how deficits affect daily life. The answers to these questions are used in conjunction with test results to develop compensatory strategies for these situations as well as strategies that can be generalized to all aspects of daily life. The treatment plan includes education of the patient and family about the nature of the deficits and why it adversely affects them and development of compensatory strategies and therapeutic activities to target specific difficulties.

Memory and New Learning

Memory and new learning are especially problematic when it is difficult to quickly determine main ideas and filter distracting versus relevant details. As a result, memory acquisition, storage, and retrieval become inefficient. Treatment targets memory deficits via extensive practice in synthesizing main elements and filtering out extraneous details with increasingly complex material. This skill is also effective for learning to take effective notes. The person's ability and willingness to take structured and consistent notes during treatment and at home have been observed in clinical practice as one of the best strategies for improved spontaneous recall and follow-through. It is vital to develop a consistent system that uses a single location for notes and includes prompts to write and review the notes. A commercial day planner is a simple, inexpensive, and effective strategy for this system. It is also important to break new information into smaller units to be rehearsed and practiced, then summarized and noted. This strategy maximizes the chance that it will be stored and ready for later retrieval, before moving on to new material.

Speed of Information Processing

Reduced speed of information processing can also adversely affect daily activities on many levels, including in conversation, when following directions, and mentally juggling ideas. Strategies are taught to slow the speed of incoming information by taking notes and asking clarifying questions in conversations or lectures. Receiving the same information in multiple complementary modalities (visual, auditory, written) seems to be beneficial to maximizing accuracy of input and retention. For example, a person may request an e-mail follow-up of quickly presented verbal auditory instructions to reinforce memory and understanding and maximize the chances for successful follow-through. It is also not an incidental factor for the person facing new information to enter the situation prepared (eg, to heighten their awareness of the techniques that they need to succeed and when to use them, to put extra effort into focused attention, to try to make use of settings that minimize distractions and tools that maximize understanding).

Attention

The ability to shift attention without succumbing to internal or external distractions is a significant challenge. Many people with MS describe this phenomenon as "going down the rabbit hole" and then losing track of what was important. The first line of defense is to assess the environment to see what kinds of distractions are present so that those can then be minimized. Distractions can be visual, auditory, or internal. Simple strategies include wearing headphones or earplugs to decrease nonrelevant auditory distractions. For visual distractions, an environment can be created with limited clutter and fewer people present. To manage internal distractions, a person can quickly jot down intrusive ideas as they come to mind if these are items that should not be forgotten, rather than shifting attention to the new thought. It is also helpful to have a written plan for the day to focus on completing a particular set of tasks, few in number and manageable in size. Cognitive rehabilitation treatment also helps the person identify those tasks that are performed routinely, either at home or at work, and to develop a plan that helps decrease the number of times when shifts in attention are required. An example of this strategy is to check e-mail only at scheduled times and only for a certain period, rather than having alerts sound throughout the day that require the person to shift attention at every announcement.

Executive Functions: Use of Structure and Routines

Structure is a critical component to successfully maintaining attention and completing tasks in a day. Often, the person with MS is completely overwhelmed by the number and complexity of the tasks that they must complete. They may also believe they have no control over their schedule. However, by creating some structure, it is easier to stay on task. Because it is difficult for someone with MS to predict how their symptoms will affect them each day, the schedule has to have some flexibility. Helping the person develop daily and weekly anchors (eg, routine scheduled tasks such as the morning get-ready process or a regular exercise time with activities that can be modified if needed) and a time to plan each day is more effective than a rigid weekly schedule that was developed a priori to complete tasks. It is also helpful to schedule blocks of time to work without interruption. Using consistent routines facilitates increased attention and follow-through of tasks as well as providing effective structure to the day/week. These routines are more successful if they are sequence based rather than time based, because of the variability of physical symptoms (eg, fatigue).

Executive Functions: Techniques for Project Completion

People with MS are frequently unable to complete projects because they do not know how best to start or become distracted in carrying out the project. In treatment, the clinician helps develop a system to plan the steps in the projects, put those steps in order, and then schedule a time to complete each of the steps. Additional strategies to prompt the person to initiate the task or to pause and assess how they are progressing may also need to be taught. Use of timers or posting and checking the plan are suggestions for additional prompts. Another component of difficulty with project completion is time management. People with MS sometimes report a diminished or absent sense of elapsed time, or that tasks take longer as a result of fatigue. Further, they may be calculating their estimates of how long a project will take based on premorbid experience and speed of performance, without taking into consideration the effects of MS. In addition, physical limitations, heightened distractibility, and memory retrieval disruptions can all contribute to more time needed. We encourage patients to double or triple the amount of estimated time needed to complete each step in the project. If they finish more quickly than estimated, that is bonus time, rather than having the stress of approaching deadlines that are impossible to meet given inaccurate planning.

Education and Awareness

The importance of the person's awareness of deficits (as well as of residual strengths) was alluded to earlier. An important aspect of overall neurorehabilitation (of which cognitive retraining/cognitive rehabilitation is a fundamental component) revolves around on-going education. By helping the person understand the relationship between specific kinds of cognitive impairments and their functional difficulties, they are better able to implement appropriate strategies. This kind of education can also facilitate ability to generalize strategies to additional tasks. By understanding the cause of the problem, (ie, why the difficulty manifests in the ways that it does), the person is less likely to be overwhelmed by it and more likely to be empowered to take control of the problem and its negative repercussions.

Unique Challenges for Cognitive Function in MS

There are particular challenges to providing treatment to people with MS, which are not typical of other forms of acquired brain injury. One of the most pressing issues for people with MS is the variability in functional deficits that they may experience day to day related to fatigue, pain, or other sensory, motor, and physical symptoms. The combination, intensity, and unpredictability of symptoms can also be demoralizing from a psychological stand-point, leading to reactive emotional distress, which can aggravate the negative impact of residual neurologic difficulties. As a function of these problems in day-to-day variability, people with MS need some degree of flexibility in their schedules as well as time for scheduled rest breaks to pace energy expenditure.

Generalization and Follow-Through with Strategies at Home

Another challenge for people with compromise in executive functions is to achieve a level of basic organization in one's home or work life to make most effective use of all strategies. Working together to identify a family member, friend, or professional organizer who can assist in creating a work or home environment where visual and auditory distractions are minimized and a truly sustainable functional organizational system is in place may be necessary for application and maintenance of strategies. Individuals with MS, especially given the progressive nature of the illness, also benefit from a return to treatment periodically to review relevant strategies, modify them further for current needs, and identify new compensatory techniques as appropriate.

SUMMARY

It is our observation over a combined 70 years or more of experience in neurorehabilitation that the cognitive rehabilitation specialist is the instrument of change for improved function in people with cognitive deficits caused by neurologic injury or illness. Although computer-based tasks can be fun, or allow practice with word games or other academic skills, unless they translate into practical applications for improved day-to-day function, they are not the best use of the person's time and resource to achieve specific real-world improvements in cognitive performance.

REFERENCES

1. Rao SM, Leo GJ, Bernardin L, et al. Cognitive dysfunction in multiple sclerosis. I. Frequency, patterns, and prediction. Neurology 1991;41(5):685–91.
2. Rao SM, Leo GJ, Ellington L, et al. Cognitive dysfunction in multiple sclerosis. II. Impact on employment and social functioning. Neurology 1991;41(5):692–6.
3. Arnett PA, Rao SM, Grafman J, et al. Executive functions in multiple sclerosis: an analysis of temporal ordering, semantic encoding, and planning abilities. Neuropsychology 1997;11(4):535–44.
4. Fischer JS. Cognitive impairment in multiple sclerosis. In: Cook SD, editor. Handbook of multiple sclerosis. 3rd edition. New York: Marcel Dekker; 2001. p. 233–55.
5. D'Esposito M, Ohishi K, Thompson H, et al. Working memory impairments in multiple sclerosis: evidence from a dual task paradigm. Neuropsychology 1996;10: 51–6.
6. Beatty WW, Goodkin DE, Monson N, et al. Cognitive disturbances in patients with relapsing remitting multiple sclerosis. Arch Neurol 1989;46:1113–9.
7. Beatty WW. Multiple sclerosis. In: Adams RL, Parsons OA, Gulbertson JL, et al, editors. Neuropsychology for clinical practice: etiology, assessment, and treatment of common neurological disorders. Washington, DC: American Psychological Association; 1996. p. 225–42.
8. DeLuca J, Gaudino EA, Diamond BJ, et al. Acquisition and storage deficits in multiple sclerosis. J Clin Exp Neuropsychol 1998;20:376–90.
9. Pepping M, Ehde D. Neuropsychological evaluation and treatment of multiple sclerosis: the importance of a neuro-rehabilitation focus. Phys Med Rehabil Clin N Am 2005;16(2):411–36.
10. Huijbregts SC, Kalkers NF, de Sonneville LM, et al. Cognitive impairment and decline in different MS subtypes. J Neurol Sci 2006;245:187–94.
11. Potogas C, Giogkaraki E, Koutsis G, et al. Cognitive impairment in different MS subtypes and clinically isolated syndromes. J Neurol Sci 2008;267(1–2):100–6.
12. DeLuca J, Chelune GJ, Tulsky DS, et al. Is speed of processing or working memory the primary information-processing deficit in multiple sclerosis? J Clin Exp Neuropsychol 2004;26(4):550–62.
13. Trapp B, Nave KA. Multiple sclerosis: an immune or neurodegenerative disorder. Annu Rev Neurosci 2008;31:247–69.
14. Hohol MJ, Guttmann CR, Oray J, et al. Serial neuropsychological assessment and magnetic resonance imaging analysis in multiple sclerosis. Arch Neurol 1997;54:1018–25.
15. O'Connor P. Key issues in the diagnosis and treatment of multiple sclerosis: an overview. Neurology 2002;59(Suppl 3):S1–3.
16. Vigeveno RM, Wiebenga OT, Wattjes MP, et al. Shifting imaging targets in multiple sclerosis: from inflammation to neurodegeneration. J Magn Reson Imaging 2012; 36:1–19.
17. Rudick R, Fisher E, Lee JC, et al. Use of the brain parenchymal fraction to measure whole brain atrophy in relapsing remitting MS. Neurology 1999;53:1698–704.
18. Chelune GJ, Stott H, Pinkston JB. Multiple sclerosis. In: Morgan J, Ricker J, editors. Textbook of clinical neuropsychology. New York: Taylor & Francis; 2008. p. 599–615.
19. Fazekas F, Barkhof F, Filippi M, et al. The contribution of magnetic resonance imaging to the diagnosis of multiple sclerosis. Neurology 1999;53:448–56.
20. Foong J, Rozewicz L, Quaghebeur G, et al. Executive function in multiple sclerosis: the role of frontal lobe pathology. Brain 1997;120(Pt 1):15–26.

21. Wallin MT, Wilken JA, Kane R. Cognitive dysfunction in multiple sclerosis: assessment, imaging and risk factors. J Rehabil Res Dev 2006;43(1):63–72.

22. Rao SM, Leo GJ, Haughton VM, et al. Correlation of magnetic resonance imaging with neuropsychological testing in multiple sclerosis. Neurology 1989;39:161–6.

23. Rovaris M, Filippi M, Minicucci L, et al. Cortical/subcortical disease burden and cognitive impairment in patients with multiple sclerosis. AJNR Am J Neuroradiol 2000;21:402–8.

24. Moriarty DM, Blackshaw AJ, Talbot PR, et al. Memory dysfunction in multiple sclerosis corresponds to juxtacortical lesion load on fast fluid-attenuated inversion-recovery MR images. AJNR Am J Neuroradiol 1999;20(10):1956–62.

25. Bermel RA, Bakshi R, Tjoa C, et al. Bicaudate ratio as a magnetic resonance imaging marker of brain atrophy in multiple sclerosis. Arch Neurol 2002;59:275–80.

26. Benedict RH, Bruce JM, Dwyer MG, et al. Neocortical atrophy, third ventricular width, and cognitive dysfunction in multiple sclerosis. Arch Neurol 2006;63:1301–6.

27. Benedict RH, Weinstock-Guttman B, Fishman I, et al. Prediction of neuropsychological impairment in multiple sclerosis: comparison of conventional magnetic resonance imaging measures of atrophy and lesion burden. Arch Neurol 2004;61:226–30.

28. Fischer E, Benedict RH. Correlation of cognitive impairment and thalamic atrophy in MS: for men only? Neurology 2012;79:1748–9.

29. Schoonheim MM, Popescu V, Rueda Lopes FC, et al. Subcortical atrophy and cognition: sex effects in multiple sclerosis. Neurology 2012;79:1754–61.

30. Benedict RH, Fischer JS, Archibald CJ, et al. Minimal neuropsychological assessment of MS patients: a consensus approach. Clin Neuropsychol 2002;16(3):381–97.

31. Benedict RH, Hussein S, Englert J, et al. Cortical atrophy and personality in multiple sclerosis. Neuropsychology 2008;22(4):432–41.

32. Ben-Yishay Y, Diller L. Cognitive remediation in traumatic brain injury: update and issues. Arch Phys Med Rehabil 1993;74:204–13.

33. Cicerone KD, Dahlberg C, Malec JF, et al. Evidence-based cognitive rehabilitation: updated review of the literature from 1998 through 2002. Arch Phys Med Rehabil 2005;86(8):1681–92.

34. Mattioli FF, Stampatori CC, Bellomi FF, et al. Neuropsychological rehabilitation in adult multiple sclerosis. Neurol Sci 2010;31:271–4.

35. Rosti-Otajärvi EM, Hämäläinen PI. Neuropsychological rehabilitation for multiple sclerosis. Cochrane Database Syst Rev 2011;(11):CD009131. http://dx.doi.org/10.1002/14651858.CD009131.pub2.

36. Flavia M, Stampatori C, Zanotti D, et al. Efficacy and specificity of intensive cognitive rehabilitation of attention and executive functions in multiple sclerosis. J Neurol Sci 2010;288(1–2):101–5.

37. O'Brien AR, Chiaravalloti N, Goverover Y, et al. Evidenced-based cognitive rehabilitation for persons with multiple sclerosis: a review of the literature. Arch Phys Med Rehabil 2008;89(4):761–9.

38. National Multiple Sclerosis Society. Expert opinion paper: assessment and management of cognitive impairment in multiple sclerosis. New York: The Multiple Sclerosis Society; 2006.

39. Kennedy MR, Coelho C, Turkstra L, et al. Intervention for executive functions after traumatic brain injury: a systematic review, meta-analysis and clinical recommendations. Neuropsychol Rehabil 2008;18(3):257–99.

40. Ehlardt L, Sohlberg MM, Kennedy MR, et al. Evidence-based practice guidelines for instructing individuals with acquired memory impairments: what have we learned in the past 20 years? Neuropsychol Rehabil 2008;18(3):300–42.
41. Sohlberg MM, Kennedy MR, Avery J, et al. Evidence based practice for the use of external aids as a memory rehabilitation technique. J Med Speech Lang Pathol 2007;15(1):xv–li.
42. Dahlberg CA, Cusick CP, Hawley LA, et al. Treatment efficacy of social communication skills training after traumatic brain injury: a randomized treatment and deferred treatment controlled trial. Arch Phys Med Rehabil 2007;88(12):1561–73.
43. Cicerone K, Dahlberg C, Kalmar K, et al. Evidence-based cognitive rehabilitation: recommendations for clinical practice. Arch Phys Med Rehabil 2000;81: 1596–615.

Bladder Management in Multiple Sclerosis

Claire C. Yang, MD

KEYWORDS

- Bladder • Urinary tract • Neurogenic bladder • Treatment

KEY POINTS

- The goals of treatment of patients with multiple sclerosis (MS) and neurogenic bladders are to preserve renal function, achieve social continence, and to minimize urinary tract complications.
- Treatments should be tailored to a patient's functional capacity.
- Initial assessment and treatment of the neurogenic bladder can be done by the primary MS provider.

INTRODUCTION

Persons with multiple sclerosis (MS) frequently experience sequelae of the disease in the urinary tract. The severity of the urologic symptoms can be highly variable but generally speaking, the more disabled a person is from MS, the more likely neurologic bladder dysfunction is present.[1,2] Because individuals do not uniformly feel bothered to the same degree given a particular set of lower urinary tract symptoms, the reporting of bladder symptoms by persons with MS is also highly variable. Quality of life issues notwithstanding, poor bladder management can result in urinary incontinence, urinary tract infections (UTIs) (which may provoke MS exacerbations), kidney and bladder stone formation, and loss of renal function. Thus, proper management of the neurogenic bladder is of utmost importance.

The goals of treatment of patients with MS and neurogenic bladders are to (1) preserve renal function, (2) achieve social continence, and (3) minimize urinary tract complications. This article reviews the basic principles and therapeutic options in the management of the neurogenic bladder due to MS, directed primarily to the nonurology provider. There are several published literature reviews and guidelines on bladder management in MS,[1,3–6] and although they contain recurring themes, there is no clear consensus on a treatment algorithm.[6] This article incorporates many of the recommendations, within the context of the author's extensive experience of providing urologic care for patients with MS.

Disclosures: None.
Department of Urology, University of Washington, Box 356510, Seattle, WA 98195-6510, USA
E-mail address: cyang@u.washington.edu

Phys Med Rehabil Clin N Am 24 (2013) 673–686
http://dx.doi.org/10.1016/j.pmr.2013.06.004
1047-9651/13/$ – see front matter Published by Elsevier Inc.

LOWER URINARY TRACT ANATOMY AND PHYSIOLOGY
Anatomy

The lower urinary tract is composed of the bladder, which includes the internal sphincter, external sphincter, and urethra (**Fig. 1**). The bladder is a hollow muscular reservoir within the pelvis. It is composed of interconnecting smooth muscle cells interspersed with elastin and collagen fibers and lined with transitional cell epithelium. The bladder is immediately posterior to the symphysis pubis. The posterior wall and dome of the bladder abut the uterus in women, and in men the ano-rectum is posterior to the bladder. The dome of the bladder is covered by peritoneum, so the bladder is closely related to the sigmoid colon and small intestines. The ureters enter the bladder on its posteroinferior surface. The muscle fibers of the bladder condense into a funnel-like structure at the base forming the bladder neck, also known as the internal sphincter. The structure is not a true circular sphincter, but a thickening of muscle as the bladder transitions into the urethra.

The female urethra is approximately 4 cm long and lies beneath the pubic symphysis, adjoining the anterior vaginal wall. Midway along the urethra is a true sphincter composed of striated muscle, the external sphincter. It is part of the pelvic floor musculature and surrounds the middle third of the urethra in women. In men, the urethra extends out from the internal sphincter and traverses the prostate gland, which is approximately 3 to 4 cm in length. Immediately distal to the prostate gland is the point at which the external sphincter surrounds the male urethra. Past the external sphincter, the urethra continues through the penile shaft to the urinary meatus at the glans penis.

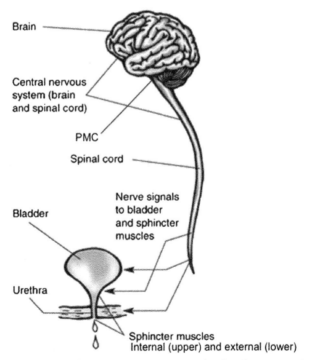

Fig. 1. Lower urinary tract and its innervation. See text for details. Lower urinary tract function is highly dependent on an intact nervous system. The detrusor reflex is coordinated in the pontine micturition center (PMC). MS lesions in the brain and spinal cord can result in neurogenic bladder and sphincter dysfunction.

The lower urinary tract is innervated by components of both the somatic and autonomic nervous systems (see **Fig. 1**). The bladder receives its motor innervation through the autonomic pelvic nerves, which are derived from spinal segments S2–S4, with most of the innervation from S3. The bladder neck or internal sphincter is innervated by the hypogastric nerves, which are derived from spinal segments T11-L1. The external sphincter is the only structure in the lower urinary tract to receive somatic motor innervation, and this is mediated through a branch of the perineal nerve, the second segment of the pudendal nerve. Its fibers are derived from spinal segments S2–S4. The sensory fibers for the structures of the lower urinary tract follow the same tracts as their respective motor fibers.

Physiology

Lower urinary tract function is a complex system of reflexes, involving the bladder, internal sphincter, external sphincter, urethra, peripheral nerves, spinal cord, and brain. Neurologic diseases such as multiple sclerosis can result in pathology at any level along the neuraxis and affect the interaction of these reflexes, causing lower urinary tract dysfunction.

In most healthy humans, both kidneys produce urine that drains through the ureters and accumulates in the bladder. The normal function of the bladder is to store urine until it has reached appropriate capacity and is socially acceptable to evacuate. Urine storage is accomplished at low pressures because the bladder wall contains elastin, which allows it to stretch without subsequent increase in pressure. Typical adult bladder capacity is approximately 300 to 500 mL.

The internal sphincter, or bladder neck, remains closed during bladder filling, and the closure is mediated through a constant sympathetic discharge via the hypogastric nerves. Thus, the internal sphincter's function is purely involuntary. The external sphincter, composed of striated muscle, also maintains a resting tone. It reflexively contracts to maintain continence during periods of increased intra-abdominal pressure and also contracts under voluntary control to shut off the urinary stream or to inhibit urinary urgency.

The detrusor reflex (also known as the micturition reflex) consists of an afferent arm, a central nervous system (CNS) nucleus, and an efferent arm. As the bladder fills, its visceral afferents travel through the pelvic nerves innervating the bladder, ascending through the spinal cord to the pontine micturition center (CNS nucleus) in the midbrain. As bladder volume approaches capacity, the sensation of fullness reaches consciousness, which prompts the individual to seek an appropriate environment in which to urinate. During this time of bladder filling, inhibitory signals from the frontal cortex project on to the pontine micturition center, which prevent the detrusor reflex from occurring. When bladder capacity is reached and is socially acceptable to evacuate urine, the inhibitory signals are withdrawn and a detrusor contraction is initiated at the pontine micturition center. An efferent response travels through the spinal cord and pelvic nerves, and a detrusor contraction occurs. The contraction is coordinated with the opening of the internal and external sphincters to allow free egress of urine from the bladder. A normal detrusor contraction of adequate strength and duration empties the bladder completely in one coordinated and sustained contraction. After urine evacuation, the sphincters return to their closed state and the cycle resumes.

Pathophysiology

Lower urinary tract dysfunction in MS can manifest in one or more of 4 possible physiologic disruptions, depending on the location of neurologic damage or demyelination.

Loss of sensation

If the sensory fibers carrying messages of bladder distention to the CNS are disrupted by demyelination, then the pontine micturition center does not receive adequate stimulus with which to initiate a detrusor contraction. Persons with loss of bladder sensation experience urinary retention or incomplete bladder emptying.

Loss of cortical inhibition of the detrusor reflex

This is the most common manifestation of bladder dysfunction in MS.[1] Because of MS lesions, the inhibition of the detrusor reflex by the frontal cortex is lost or impaired, resulting in bladder contractions with limited volitional control. Patients experience urinary urgency (strong sensation to urinate, typically as the bladder starts to contract), frequency (frequent voiding of small urine volumes), and urge incontinence (urine leak as a result of an inability to inhibit the detrusor reflex). This type of bladder activity is also known as "overactive bladder" and resembles the bladder of a child before toilet training; there is an impaired or absent cortical control over the detrusor reflex.

Inefficient bladder contractility

As described earlier, the healthy bladder empties regularly and efficiently, in a coordinated, sustained contraction. With significant spinal cord disease or injury, the bladder contraction is not of adequate contraction strength or duration to empty the bladder in a single coordination, likely as a result of incoordination with the pontine micturition center. What results is a partially emptied bladder with each void, with varying degrees of urinary retention.

Bladder outlet obstruction

One form of bladder outlet obstruction exclusive to patients with spinal cord disease or injury (including patients with MS) is the loss of coordination between bladder and sphincter activity. If the urinary sphincters, which are closed during filling, do not relax and open before bladder contraction, then there is a functional obstruction to bladder drainage. This incoordination of the sphincters and bladder is known as detrusor-sphincter dyssynergia and results in urinary hesitancy, a sense of incomplete emptying, and urinary retention. With the absence of detrusor-sphincter dyssynergia, women with MS rarely experience bladder outlet obstruction. Men can have obstruction as they age, with an enlarging prostate gland impinging on the bladder neck, causing lower urinary tract symptoms.

NEUROGENIC BLADDER MANAGEMENT
Principles

There are several principles of bladder management that serve to guide treatment decision making, to reach the goals of renal preservation, achievement of social continence, and minimization of lower urinary tract complications. MS health care providers should keep in mind these general concepts as they develop individualized plans of care with their patients.

1. *The bladder should empty regularly and efficiently.* This is the primary principle to adhere to, as bladder emptying determines the frequency and severity of lower urinary symptoms and morbidity, which ultimately can affect renal function. The healthy adult bladder in an asymptomatic person empties completely approximately 4 to 8 times every 24 hours, depending on fluid intake. Infrequent and inefficient emptying can result in lower urinary tract symptoms, infections, and incontinence. If a patient cannot spontaneously and efficiently void, the use of catheters can overcome bladder emptying failure.

2. *Bladder management should be appropriate to functional capacity and should proceed from the least invasive to most invasive techniques, and least complicated to most complicated.* Each patient's cognitive and physical condition will dictate the optimal method for bladder management. Given the progressive nature of MS, these conditions can change with time, and so bladder management must accommodate those changes. Methods to manage the neurogenic bladder can range from very simple behavioral modifications to extensive surgical reconstruction of the urinary tract. Providers and patients should realize that complex bladder management techniques may not be appropriate for patients who are significantly impaired or for patients who have rapidly progressive disease.

3. *Bladder emptying should be independent of caregivers.* This is a corollary to the principle discussed earlier. Many patients who are debilitated are unable to empty their bladders spontaneously and thus require catheterization. In an effort to avoid chronic indwelling catheterization, some patients are placed on an intermittent catheterization program, performed by caregivers. Although this program may well decrease the risks of chronic catheterization, it creates an unsustainable management plan, whereby a caregiver is required to be present 24 hours per day. In situations where such care is available, typically the caregivers are not the same personnel from day to day, and the risks of UTIs and urethral injury due to inexperienced caregivers far outweigh the risks of chronic catheterization. If patients are in an environment with limited numbers of caregivers (eg, family members), the burden of care can be overwhelming.

4. *Effective bowel management is critical to effective bladder management.* Because the innervation to the bladder and urethra neuroanatomically overlap with the innervation of the anorectum, the optimization of bladder management necessarily depends on the optimization of bowel care. Regular, efficient emptying of the rectum minimizes the risk of UTIs, facilitates bladder emptying, and improves quality of life.[7] Bowel function can also be affected by lower urinary tract management. For example, many medications used to treat lower urinary tract symptoms (eg, anticholinergic medications) have constipation as a side effect, and so bowel care should be optimized before starting these medications.

5. *There are sex differences in neurogenic bladder management.* Although the urinary tract physiology of both women and men are the same, the anatomic differences translate into practical considerations when determining an optimal bladder management plan. For example, women who wear chronic indwelling urethral catheters for many years are at high risk for urethral erosion (which results in urine leak around the catheter) particularly if they are post-menopausal. Women who perform intermittent catheterization must be able to transfer to a toilet and catheterize themselves without being able to visualize their urethras, whereas men are able to catheterize and drain urine into a urinal without necessarily needing to transfer, and they are able to visualize their urethral meatus for self-catheterization. Older men (eg, aged >55–60 years) with urinary symptoms may have an enlarged prostate factoring into their pathophysiology, whereas older women may have pelvic floor complications (eg, bladder prolapse) contributing to theirs.

Techniques

There are a large number of treatment options for the MS patient with neurogenic bladder symptoms, ranging from the simple behavioral modifications to the complex urinary tract reconstruction. The most commonly used methods are outlined in **Box 1** and arranged in ascending order with respect to invasiveness (NB, the list does not encompass all possible bladder management options). When considering

---

Box 1
Bladder management techniques

1. Behavioral modifications
   a. Timed voiding
   b. Fluid restriction
   c. Biofeedback and physical therapy
   d. Valsalva and crede maneuver
   d. External collection devices
2. Medications
   a. Anticholinergics
   b. Tricyclic antidepressants
   c. Botulinum toxin
   d. Desmopressin
   e. Effects of polypharmacy
   f. Dietary supplements and herbal preparations
3. Catheterization
   a. Chronic indwelling
   b. Clean intermittent
4. Lower urinary tract reconstruction
   a. Urethral sling
   b. Neuromodulation
   c. Bladder reconstruction
   d. Urinary diversion/ileal conduit

---

these options for a particular patient, providers should keep in mind the treatment principles outlined in the last section. The following descriptions of the techniques are meant to provide an overview and not as an instructional guide.

Behavioral modifications

As the least invasive and oftentimes the easiest therapies to institute, behavioral modifications are the first-line options in managing neurogenic bladder symptoms. To better direct the behavioral modifications, a very instructive exercise for patients is to have them carry out a diary of their fluid intake and voiding output. Using an hourly chart, patients document volume of fluid consumed and volume voided (or evacuated, if using intermittent catheterization). These data can then be used to inform decisions to help manage urinary symptoms, based on when urinary volume may be affecting the patient. Three consecutive or nonconsecutive days of a diary is generally representative of the patient's schedule.

Timed voiding Timed voiding is voiding by a schedule, rather than when prompted to by bladder sensations. It is used in persons who have impaired bladder sensation (but retained contractility), so as not to overdistend the bladder or to avoid urinary incontinence. For persons who make a large amount of fluid (eg, >800 cc) during the course of a night, a timed awakening and voiding during the middle of the night can potentially treat nighttime incontinence.

Fluid restriction Fluid restriction is the purposeful limitation of fluid intake at certain times of the day, to minimize urine production. One example is minimizing fluid intake in the evenings to treat nocturia. It also is the restriction of certain types of beverages (eg, caffeinated beverages, alcohol) to limit irritative voiding symptoms.

Biofeedback and physical therapy Biofeedback and physical therapy can be used to strengthen pelvic floor muscles that have been weakened from previous surgery or obstetric trauma. In addition, it can help to quell urinary urgency. The most recognized of the physical therapy maneuvers are the Kegel exercises. Biofeedback may involve an intravaginal or rectal electromyography device that allows the patient to have visual and auditory feedback on the efficacy of pelvic floor muscle contractions. The efficacy of biofeedback in treating bladder symptoms due to MS is mixed.[8] Both physical therapy and biofeedback are likely only to be efficacious in persons with mild neurogenic bladder involvement; anyone with significantly compromised pelvic sensory or motor innervation will have a limited ability to comply with the therapeutic regimens.

Cognitive-based treatments including yoga[9] have been anecdotally reported to be effective in treating bladder symptoms.

Valsalva and crede maneuver These maneuvers increase intra-abdominal pressure and forcefully evacuate urine from a bladder that has inadequate contractility. The author discourages these maneuvers, as they can exacerbate existing pelvic floor weakness, with resultant pelvic organ prolapse in women. In men, inguinal hernias may result from prolonged pressure on the lower abdomen.

External urine collection devices External urine collection devices allow patients to void spontaneously, even if they are unable to toilet themselves. These collection devices include condom catheters for men (no reliable device exists for women), undergarments that mechanically draw urine away from the genitalia (eg, URINCare), and diapers or pads. Meticulous care is necessary to avoid skin irritation and breakdown with diaper use in the debilitated patient. In the highly functional patient who may have occasional urine leakage, a pad to protect undergarments is a reasonable option. There are many sizes and absorbancies of pads, to accommodate both men and women.

Medications
Many patients with neurogenic bladder dysfunction require medications to manage their bladder symptoms. Although most patients benefit symptomatically from drug treatment, medications cannot recreate a normal detrusor reflex in the neurologically impaired, and there is no medication that can improve bladder contractility. The following classes of medications are some of the more commonly used for bladder management in MS, often in combination with other techniques.

Anticholinergics These medications are the most commonly used in MS patients with bladder dysfunction, to treat the overactive bladder symptoms of urgency, frequency, and urge incontinence. Many drugs in this class are available, including oxybutynin (Ditropan), tolterodine (Detrol), solifenacin (Vesicare), darifenacin (Enablex), and trospium (Sanctura). These drugs are used to suppress detrusor contractions through anticholinergic activity and independent detrusor relaxant effects. All of these drugs can increase post-voiding residual urine volume, so clean intermittent catheterization (CIC) may be needed as an adjunctive therapy to achieve continence and efficient bladder emptying. Another prominent side effect is constipation, which many MS patients have at baseline or due to other medications. This author recommends treating constipation and having patients on a regular bowel program to generate soft, easily evacuated bowel movements at least three times a week, before starting anticholinergic medications.

Because of the multiplicity of medications in this class, it can be difficult to decide which formulation to use. It has been this author's experience that the efficacy and side effect profile of each medication is an individualized response, and a particular medication is not going to be more efficacious or have less side effects across a heterogeneous group of MS patients. In general, anticholinergic medications should be titrated to effect or side effect, that is, starting at a low dose and increasing the medication until the desired effect is achieved or an undesired side effect occurs. Short-acting preparations allow for more flexibility, with medication side effects less pronounced, since higher doses of medications can be used at times of the day when patients are more symptomatic and less medication during times of less bother. Medication cost is a significant concern for many patients, and the newer anticholinergic medications that have not gone to generic preparations can be very expensive and may not be on the formularies of many insurance programs.

For these reasons, this author starts patients on anticholinergic therapy with generic oxybutynin. The generic preparation is almost universally available, is inexpensive, and tablets can be cut in half for refined titration.

An example of a medication dosing regimen is as follows: if a patient complains of urinary urgency and frequency primarily in daytime and does not have bothersome nocturia, then a reasonable starting dose is oxybutynin 5 mg twice a day, with a dose in the morning and a dose in the afternoon. The window of efficacy is about 4 to 6 hours and then the medication can "wash out" during the evening/night hours. Oxybutynin can be titrated up in 2.5 to 5.0 mg increments. If the side effect profile is intolerable, another anticholinergic medication can be substituted.

Tricyclic antidepressants This class of medications facilitates urine storage by decreasing bladder contractility and increasing bladder outlet resistance. There are several purported mechanisms by which this is believed to occur, including anticholinergic and antihistaminic effects. Use of these medications in combination with anticholinergic agents may have an additive effect on depressing bladder contractility. The dose of tricyclic antidepressant medications for bladder symptoms is lower than that used for the treatment of depression. Examples of these drugs include imipramine (Tofranil), amitriptyline (Elavil), and nortriptyline (Pamelor). This medication class has a wide range of side effects, which are dose dependent.

Botulinum toxin A major development in the treatment of neurogenic bladder dysfunction has been the introduction of the neurotoxin, botulinum toxin (BTX), to the pharmacologic armamentarium. This agent is used to suppress detrusor contractions, thereby minimizing the symptoms of urgency, frequency, and urge incontinence. Neuromuscular blockade via inhibition of acetylcholine release with subsequent muscle paralysis is the most acknowledged mechanism that is attributed to BTX,[10] and it is also believed to have some effect on sensory fibers as well. It was approved by the Food and Drug Administration (FDA) in 2011 for the treatment of neurogenic bladder dysfunction, after many studies demonstrated its efficacy in a wide range of patients, including MS.[11,12] The use of BTX has significantly reduced the need for major lower urinary tract reconstructive surgery, to maintain a compliant, stable bladder. It is administered through an injection needle modified for a cystoscope (**Fig. 2**) and is performed as a brief clinic or outpatient surgical procedure. The efficacy of the BTX wears off with time, requiring reinjection every 6 to 12 months. The primary side effect of the treatment is urinary retention, and patients should be

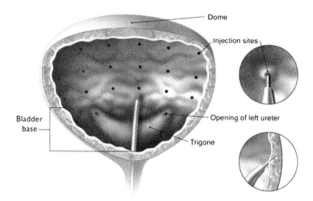

Fig. 2. Demonstration of intradetrusor injection of BTX to treat overactive bladder symptoms. A long needle is introduced through a cystoscope to inject small aliquots of BTX throughout the bladder. (*From* Fowler CJ, Auerbach S, Ginsberg D. OnabotulinumtoxinA improves health-related quality of life in patients with urinary incontinence due to idiopathic overactive bladder: a 36-week, double-blind, placebo-controlled, randomized, dose-ranging trial. Eur Urol 2012;62(1):148–57; with permission.)

prepared to perform CIC post-operatively, even if they are voiding spontaneously before the procedure.

Desmopressin Desmopressin (DDAVP) is a synthetic version of the hormone vasopressin. It acts to decrease urine formation and is used to treat daytime or nighttime urinary frequency. A meta-analysis done on its use in MS patients with bladder symptoms shows desmopressin has a moderate effect on the number of voids during the day or during the night over a period of 6 hours after taking the drug.[13] However, its efficacy and any potential electrolyte abnormalities with long-term use are not known.

Effects of polypharmacy Poor bladder function, in the form of impaired bladder sensation and diminished contractile strength, can be a result of medications used by MS patients for the management of nonbladder-related MS symptoms. The medications' side effects are a result of primary medication use, or as a result of pharmaceutical combinations. The classes of medications that can impair bladder function include the following: anticholinergics, antianxiolytics, muscle relaxants, narcotics, antidepressants, and antiepileptics (such as those used for the treatment of chronic pain). The author does not advocate eliminating medications for the optimization of bladder function, but providers should be aware of the possible effects of multiple medications on bladder function.

Dietary supplements and herbal preparations A variety of dietary supplements and herbal preparations claim to have potential benefits for MS patients. With few exceptions, the effectiveness of these remedies for treating MS symptoms has not been evaluated in controlled trials. Dietary supplements and herbal preparations can have potentially serious side effects and some can interfere or interact with prescription medications.

Catheter drainage
For persons in urinary retention, catheter drainage effectively drains the bladder of urine. Modern management of catheter and bladder care has allowed patients requiring catheter drainage to maintain a healthy lifestyle for many decades. Although

there are more complications of chronic catheterization compared with CIC, chronic catheterization in the debilitated patient allows for efficient and constant emptying of the bladder, thereby minimizing the risks of renal damage.

Chronic (indwelling) catheterization This is the only option for adequate bladder emptying in debilitated persons with urinary retention. An indwelling catheter can be placed per urethra or as a surgically placed suprapubic tube. There is no difference in the UTI rate with either catheter position, nor is there any difference based on the material of the catheter. There are some advantages to suprapubic tube placement, including ease of catheter exchange, patient comfort, and accommodation for sexual activity. Women who are chronically catheterized for years (particularly following menopause) have a very high incidence of urethral erosion, which will require surgical closure of the bladder neck and suprapubic tube placement if problematic incontinence results. The author thus advocates early suprapubic tube placement in women who are bound to indwelling catheter drainage.

Clean intermittent catheterization CIC is a technique for bladder emptying, without using an indwelling catheter. CIC is often used in combination with medications, typically from the anticholinergic class, to suppress bladder contractions and prevent leakage in between catheterizations. As noted earlier, bladder paralysis via intradetrusor BTX injections also helps to maintain bladder compliance and minimize bladder overactivity. The method of catheterization is clean, not sterile, because urethral colonization of bacteria will always result in inoculation of the bladder by catheterization. However, an atraumatic technique and regular, efficient emptying of the bladder (eg, every 4–6 hours or 4–5 times per day) will minimize the likelihood of urinary infection.

CIC requires that the patient be cognitively functional to maintain a catheterization schedule, because an inadequate frequency of catheterization (eg, twice a day) will result in sequela such as UTIs. Adequate hand dexterity is needed to pass the catheter per urethra. In addition, women performing CIC should have enough mobility to transfer onto a toilet. CIC should be performed by the patient, and not rely on others to do it, again to minimize the sequela of infrequent catheterization or traumatic catheterization by caregivers. Catheterization does not require patients to be home-bound; it can be easily performed in public restrooms and while traveling.

LOWER URINARY TRACT RECONSTRUCTION

Surgical procedures on the lower urinary tract should generally be considered only after less invasive management techniques have been proved unsuccessful. The following are some of the more commonly performed reconstructive operations that have been used to treat urinary tract complications of MS.

Urethral Sling

Urethral sling procedures are performed on patients with stress urinary incontinence, particularly in women. Because most persons with MS are women, there will be a certain percentage of women experiencing incontinence as a result of pelvic floor laxity, typically as a result of past pregnancies. Although sling procedures can be effective on stress incontinence, a urethral sling will not treat urge incontinence (a very frequent manifestation in MS).

Neuromodulation

Neuromodulation of the urinary tract has been gaining popularity in the last several years. It is FDA approved for the treatment of lower urinary tract symptoms refractory to medication and for the treatment of idiopathic urinary retention. The neuromodulation is achieved with the implantation of a sacral nerve root stimulator, known as sacral nerve stimulation (SNS), and its method of action is believed to be through the modulation of urinary reflexes through afferent nerve stimulation.[14] It is not a bladder motor nerve stimulation device.

The treatment of patients with MS and lower urinary tract symptoms/bladder dysfunction with SNS has been generally reported in series with heterogeneous populations with neurogenic bladders[15] or in small series dedicated to MS.[16] The reported results are typically optimistic for short-term follow-up, but long-term studies have not been reported. Several considerations have convinced this author that SNS is not an ideal treatment of MS-related bladder dysfunction:

1. The purported mechanism of SNS is through modulation of afferent nerve signals mediating lower urinary reflexes. Thus, the efficacy of SNS relies on intact innervation. It does not make sense to modulate damaged nerves; the SNS is NOT bypassing or overcoming damaged neural pathways.
2. Any procedural complication of device implantation could potentially affect the CNS and potentially exacerbate MS-related morbidity.
3. Implantation of a nerve stimulator precludes the use of magnetic resonance imaging (MRI) in many imaging centers. In a recent review of our hospital's experience, the authors identified that of 35 SNS devices explanted from a series of 155 patients with an SNS device, 16 (45%) of the devices were explanted in part due to the need for MRI.
4. Noninvasive neuromodulation techniques, such as posterior tibial nerve stimulation, may provide symptomatic relief from urinary frequency and urgency in MS patients, without the risk and costs of surgical implantation, but the literature is still immature on the topic.[17]

Bladder Reconstruction

Despite behavioral and medical therapies, the neurogenic bladder still may fail in its function to be a continent reservoir. Frequently, the bladder is labeled as "small capacity," and may have lost compliance, resulting in high bladder pressures during the filling phases. When conservative treatments fail, urologists can construct a large capacity, low-pressure urinary reservoir by placing a "patch" of bowel on a bivalved bladder (**Fig. 3**). In women, the native bladder neck may need to be closed and a continent catheterizable channel constructed, through which the patient passes a catheter to empty the reservoir. This type of reconstruction is a large and complicated operation. The patient typically needs to be fairly high functioning from a cognitive standpoint, to remember to catheterize on a regular schedule. Furthermore, she/he requires adequate manual dexterity to catheterize. With the recent introduction of intradetrusor BTX injections (see earlier discussion), the necessity for these types of bladder reconstructive procedures has dropped considerably.

Urinary Diversion/Ileal Conduit

Historically, urinary diversion through construction of an ileal conduit was a common method to avoid the morbidity of a neurogenic bladder. This operation diverts urine from the bladder by surgically rerouting both ureters into a segment of ileum taken out of continuity of the gastrointestinal tract. The ileal conduit then drains urine through a stoma on the abdominal wall (**Fig. 4**). With the development of better bladder management, this option has not been used with the same frequency as in years past. The

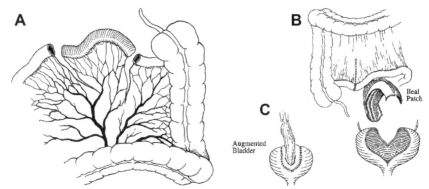

Fig. 3. Construction of bladder augmentation. (*A*) A segment of distal ileum is isolated, keeping its blood supply intact within the mesentery. (*B*) The ileal segment is opened on its antimesenteric border, creating a bowel "patch." (*C*) The patch is attached onto the bivalved bladder, thereby increasing bladder capacity and dissipating any bladder contractions.

morbidity of the operation as well as the high incidence of hydronephrosis and electrolyte imbalances are known long-term complications of ileal conduit formation.

INITIAL CLINIC-BASED MANAGEMENT OF NEUROGENIC BLADDER IN MS

Because of the high frequency of bladder complaints in persons with MS,[2] all patients should be queried about their bladder function by their MS care provider. If there are bothersome complaints, the initial management can be performed by within the physiatry, neurology, or primary care clinic. A urology consultation can be obtained when initial management does not appear to be effective, or if there are conditions, for example, urinary tract stones or hematuria, which require further evaluation.

Taking a careful history documenting urinary symptoms, any urologic or urogynecologic operations, and bowel habits is an excellent start (**Fig. 5**). An uncomplicated genitourinary examination can be performed, examining the abdomen, lower extremities,

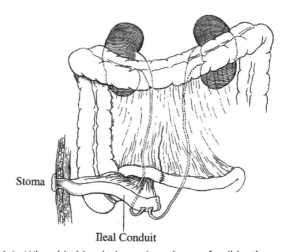

Fig. 4. Ileal conduit. When bladder drainage is no longer feasible, the same type of bowel segment from **Fig. 3** can be used to drain urine through a stoma on the abdominal wall.

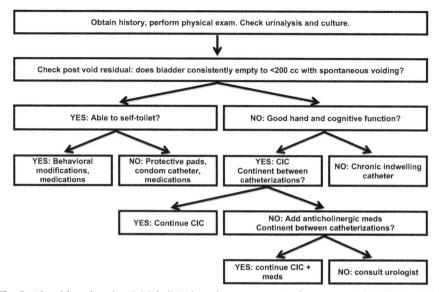

Fig. 5. Algorithm showing initial clinic-based management of neurogenic bladder in MS.

and external genitalia. Significant neurologic impairment of the lower extremities is highly predictive of genitourinary dysfunction[18] due to the proximity of neurologic pathways. Symptoms suggestive of urinary tract infection in a person who is not chronically catheterized merit a urinalysis and urine culture on initial evaluation.

A post-void residual measurement, which can be measured with an office-based, portable ultrasonic device, is an invaluable piece of data. The efficacy with which the bladder empties determines which path of treatment to pursue. As a general guideline, the author has arbitrarily chosen 200 cc as the point at which urinary retention becomes problematic and determines which branch of the decision tree to proceed. If a patient is able to self-toilet and empties her bladder to less than 200 cc residuals, then symptoms can be managed with behavioral modifications and medications (eg, anticholinergic medications for urgency and frequency). If the patient is unable to toilet, it is probably best to manage the bladder with external collection devices. If a patient does not void to less than 200 cc, then emptying with catheter assistance is required. A significantly disabled patient should probably be managed with a chronic catheter. A patient with good hand and cognitive function can attempt CIC. If there is still urgency/frequency or leaking in between catheterizations, anticholinergic medications can be used. If this fails, then referral to an urologist is indicated, for example, for BTX injections or other more complicated reconstructive operations.

REFERENCES

1. de Seze M, Ruffion A, Denys P, et al. The neurogenic bladder in multiple sclerosis: review of the literature and proposal of management guidelines. Mult Scler 2007;13(7):915–28.

2. Mahajan ST, Patel PB, Marrie RA. Under treatment of overactive bladder symptoms in patients with multiple sclerosis: an ancillary analysis of the NARCOMS Patient Registry. J Urol 2010;183(4):1432–7.

3. Fowler CJ, Panicker JN, Drake M, et al. A UK consensus on the management of the bladder in multiple sclerosis. J Neurol Neurosurg Psychiatry 2009;80(5): 470–7.

4. Urinary dysfunction and multiple sclerosis: evidence-based management strategies for urinary dysfunction and multiple sclerosis. Multiple Sclerosis Council practice guidelines: Washington, DC; 1999.

5. Stoffel JT. Contemporary management of the neurogenic bladder for multiple sclerosis patients. Urol Clin North Am 2010;37(4):547–57.

6. Tubaro A, Puccini F, De Nunzio C, et al. The treatment of lower urinary tract symptoms in patients with multiple sclerosis: a systematic review. Curr Urol Rep 2012; 13(5):335–42.

7. Loening-Baucke V. Urinary incontinence and urinary tract infection and their resolution with treatment of chronic constipation of childhood. Pediatrics 1997; 100(2 Pt 1):228–32.

8. Klarskov P, Heely E, Nyholdt I, et al. Biofeedback treatment of bladder dysfunction in multiple sclerosis. A randomized trial. Scand J Urol Nephrol Suppl 1994; 157:61–5.

9. Patil NJ, Nagaratna R, Garner C, et al. Effect of integrated Yoga on neurogenic bladder dysfunction in patients with multiple sclerosis-A prospective observational case series. Complement Ther Med 2012;20(6):424–30.

10. Coelho A, Dinis P, Pinto R, et al. Distribution of the high-affinity binding site and intracellular target of botulinum toxin type A in the human bladder. Eur Urol 2010;57(5):884–90.

11. Reitz A, Stohrer M, Kramer G, et al. European experience of 200 cases treated with botulinum-A toxin injections into the detrusor muscle for urinary incontinence due to neurogenic detrusor overactivity. Eur Urol 2004;45(4):510–5.

12. Karsenty G, Denys P, Amarenco G, et al. Botulinum toxin A (Botox) intradetrusor injections in adults with neurogenic detrusor overactivity/neurogenic overactive bladder: a systematic literature review. Eur Urol 2008;53(2):275–87.

13. Bosma R, Wynia K, Havlikova E, et al. Efficacy of desmopressin in patients with multiple sclerosis suffering from bladder dysfunction: a meta-analysis. Acta Neurol Scand 2005;112(1):1–5.

14. Leng WW, Chancellor MB. How sacral nerve stimulation neuromodulation works. Urol Clin North Am 2005;32(1):11–8.

15. Wallace PA, Lane FL, Noblett KL. Sacral nerve neuromodulation in patients with underlying neurologic disease. Am J Obstet Gynecol 2007;197(1):96.e91–5.

16. Minardi D, Muzzonigro G. Sacral neuromodulation in patients with multiple sclerosis. World J Urol 2012;30(1):123–8.

17. Kabay S, Kabay SC, Yucel M, et al. The clinical and urodynamic results of a 3-month percutaneous posterior tibial nerve stimulation treatment in patients with multiple sclerosis-related neurogenic bladder dysfunction. Neurourol Urodyn 2009;28(8):964–8.

18. Awad SA, Gajewski JB, Sogbein SK, et al. Relationship between neurological and urological status in patients with multiple sclerosis. J Urol 1984;132(3):499–502.

Visual Issues in Multiple Sclerosis

Courtney E. Francis, MD

KEYWORDS

- Diplopia • Fingolimod • Internuclear ophthalmoplegia • Multiple sclerosis
- Nystagmus • Optic neuritis • Optical coherence tomography

KEY POINTS

- A majority of patients with multiple sclerosis have an ophthalmic manifestation over the course of their disease.
- Optic neuritis is the most common ophthalmic manifestation of multiple sclerosis and, although typically there is spontaneous visual recovery, it is often treated with intravenous (IV) steroids.
- Patients treated with fingolimod need to be followed with serial eye examinations due to the risk of developing macular edema.

INTRODUCTION

Multiple sclerosis (MS) has several manifestations that can affect vision, with a majority of patients having a visual complaint over the course of their disease. The most common ophthalmic manifestations of MS are listed in **Box 1** and discussed later. In addition, ocular complications of treatment are considered.

OPTIC NEURITIS

Optic neuritis is the most common ophthalmic manifestation of MS, with an incidence of up to 20% of patients having optic neuritis as the initial clinical presentation of MS and up to 50% of patients having at least 1 episode over the course of their disease.[1–4]

Symptoms

Optic neuritis typically presents with acute loss of vision in 1 eye over a period of days. The vision loss is often preceded by or occurs concurrently with periorbital pain worsened with extraocular movements.[5] The pain associated with optic neuritis is likely secondary to traction on the inflamed nerve sheath by the extraocular muscles at the orbital apex and tends to improve after several days. Vision loss typically progresses over several days and then gradually improves over weeks to months.

Department of Ophthalmology, University of Washington, Box 359608, 325 9th Avenue, Seattle, WA 98104-2499, USA
E-mail address: francis3@uw.edu

Phys Med Rehabil Clin N Am 24 (2013) 687–702
http://dx.doi.org/10.1016/j.pmr.2013.06.002
1047-9651/13/$ – see front matter © 2013 Elsevier Inc. All rights reserved.

pmr.theclinics.com

Box 1
Ophthalmic manifestations of multiple sclerosis

Optic neuritis

Internuclear ophthalmoplegia

Nystagmus

Skew deviation

Cranial nerve 3, 4, or 6 palsies

Retrochiasmal visual pathway demyelination

Intermediate uveitis

The vision loss in optic neuritis can vary widely, with acuities ranging from 20/20 to no light perception.[6] Visual field defects should be present in optic neuritis but can range from small scotomata to arcuate or altitudinal defects to diffuse loss.[7] Contrast sensitivity is typically reduced and patients often report changes in color vision.

Examination Findings

On examination, a relative afferent pupillary defect should be seen in most cases. An afferent pupillary defect may not be seen if a patient has had a prior episode of optic neuritis or other optic neuropathy in the contralateral eye or has bilateral simultaneous and symmetric onset. Otherwise, the possibility of other causes of vision loss must be considered. On funduscopic examination, the optic nerve appears completely normal in approximately 65% of patients, with the remaining presenting with optic disc edema.[6] The presence of optic disc hemorrhages, high-grade disc edema, vitreous cell, or a macular star is not consistent with the diagnosis of demyelinating optic neuritis and should prompt a work-up for other causes of optic neuropathy.[8–10]

Ancillary Tests

Orbital MRI may be helpful in the diagnosis of optic neuritis in some cases. On gadolinium-enhanced, fat-suppressed T1 images, swelling and enhancement of the optic nerve may be seen approximately 90% of the time.[11–13] Because optic neuritis is a clinical diagnosis, the absence of enhancement does not rule out the diagnosis of optic neuritis, and additionally the presence of enhancement is not specific for demyelinating optic neuritis. **Fig. 1** shows an example of optic nerve enhancement on MRI in the setting of an acute episode of optic neuritis. Usually orbital imaging is reserved for atypical cases; however, as discussed later, brain MRI is an important prognostic test to assess the risk of future MS.

Optical coherence tomography (OCT) can be a useful adjunctive tool in the monitoring of optic nerve health in the setting of demyelinating optic neuritis. OCT, an optical form of ultrasound imaging, can provide high-definition cross-sectional, and 3-D imaging of the retina and optic nerve head. At initial presentation in optic neuritis, the retinal nerve fiber layer (rNFL) thickness is typically normal to slightly swollen. As visual recovery occurs, the rNFL may progressively thin, often preferentially in the temporal quadrant of the optic nerve head over a period of 6 months (**Fig. 2**).[14,15] Loss of rNFL thickness can correlate with other subjective measures of visual dysfunction, such as low-contrast acuity.[16] OCT is thought to be a useful potential adjuvant biomarker of disease activity in MS by noninvasively documenting axonal loss at the optic nerve head through serial rNFL measurements in patients.[17]

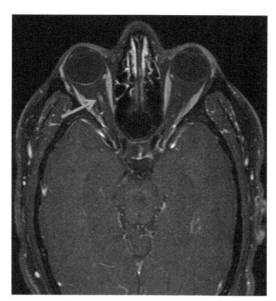

Fig. 1. An axial T1 postcontrast fat-suppressed MRI of a 29-year-old man who presented with acute loss of vision in the right eye associated with mild discomfort with extraocular movements. He was found to have 20/400 acuity in the right eye, with a right afferent pupillary defect and a normal appearance to his right optic nerve. The MRI shows enhancement within the intraorbital segment of the right optic nerve (*arrow*). He was given 3 days of IV methylprednisolone followed by a 10-day oral prednisone taper. On follow-up 2.5 months later, his visual acuity in the right eye was 20/20. His brain MRI is shown in **Fig. 4**.

Differential Diagnosis

Depending on a patient's presentation, other causes must be considered. Pain with extraocular movements can be seen with posterior scleritis and orbital myositis. Mildly decreased vision, dyschromatopsia, and an absence of disc edema can be seen in central serous retinopathy. Optic neuropathies associated with disc edema include acute anterior ischemic optic neuropathy, neuroretinitis, and other inflammatory or infectious causes of optic neuritis.[18,19] Vision loss that is bilaterally sequential and persists without improvement can be concerning for Leber hereditary optic neuropathy, a mitochondrially inherited disease that typically manifests in men in their teens to 20s. Bilateral simultaneous onset, especially when associated with longitudinally extensive transverse myelitis, should prompt further evaluation for neuromyelitis optica (NMO).[20]

Treatment and Prognosis

The landmark Optic Neuritis Treatment Trial (ONTT) generated significant information regarding the natural history of demyelinating optic neuritis by evaluating the role of steroids in the treatment of optic neuritis and the association of optic neuritis and MS.[21–25] Patients with a diagnosis of optic neuritis were randomized to receive placebo, oral prednisone, or IV methylprednisolone followed by an oral prednisone taper. Without any intervention, the vision loss secondary to optic neuritis typically spontaneously improves over the course of weeks to months, with approximately 95% of patients achieving 20/40 or better visual acuity and only 3% of patients with vision loss of 20/200 or worse.[25] More severe loss of vision at presentation is associated with worse

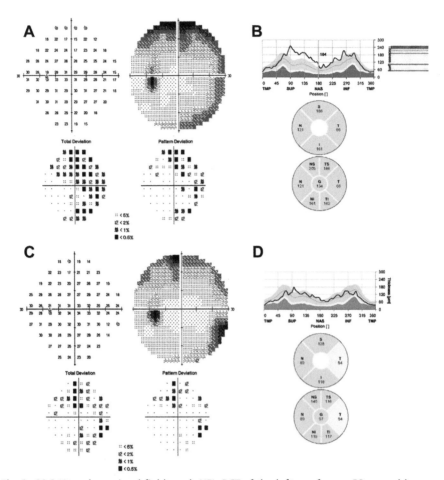

Fig. 2. 30-2 Humphrey visual fields and rNFL OCT of the left eye from a 32-year-old woman with acute optic neuritis. She reported pain with extraocular movements and decreased vision. She was found 20/20 in the left eye but with an afferent pupillary defect and dyschromatopsia. (*A*) Shows the visual field at presentation, with nasal constriction. The rNFL was swollen superiorly, as seen on OCT (*B*). On follow-up, there was some improvement on visual field testing (*C*); however, repeat OCT 1 year later revealed resolution of rNFL swelling and progressive atrophy temporally (*D*).

visual outcome. One year after an attack in optic neuritis, there was no significant difference in visual acuity, contrast sensitivity, color vision, or visual field defects between the treatment arms.[23] The administration of IV steroids, however, was well tolerated and shown to speed recovery of vision loss. Oral prednisone alone failed to improve vision and was associated with increased risk of new attacks of optic neuritis in the first 2 years (30% vs 16% in placebo and 14% in IV steroid group) and, therefore, is contraindicated in the treatment of optic neuritis.[9] Additionally, IV steroids were shown to reduce the risk of developing MS in the first 2 years (7.5% risk vs 16.5% risk in placebo).[26] The decision on whether to give IV steroids is based on the severity of vision loss, risk of developing MS, associated comorbid conditions, and patient preference. **Fig. 3** shows a Humphrey visual field of a patient at

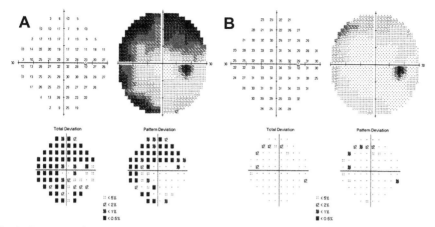

Fig. 3. 30-2 Humphrey visual fields of a patient with acute optic neuritis in the right eye. She reported pain with extraocular movements and decreased peripheral vision in the right eye. Visual acuity was 20/20 in both eyes, with a right afferent pupillary defect and normal appearing optic nerves. She was given 3 days of IV steroids. (*A*) Shows her visual field at presentation with dense constriction. (*B*) Shows her visual field 5 weeks later with significant improvement in her peripheral vision. Her MRI was consistent with MS.

presentation of acute optic neuritis in the right eye and then 5 weeks after administration of IV solumedrol.

Although most patients have significant visual recovery, residual deficits are often apparent. In the 15-year follow-up of the ONTT, 72% of affected eyes had acuities of 20/20 or better and only 2% of patients had acuities of less than or equal to 20/40 in both eyes.[27] Contrast sensitivity was not different between affected and fellow eyes but was worse in patients who went on to develop MS. Scores on the National Eye Institute Visual Function Questionnaire indicate patients with a history of optic neuritis perceive their visual function to be poorer than those who have not suffered an attack, particularly in those with reduced acuity or neurologic disability secondary to MS.

Association with Multiple Sclerosis

There is a strong association between demyelinating optic neuritis and the diagnosis of MS. From the results of the ONTT, the risk of MS in the setting of optic neuritis is now well established. The overall probability of developing MS after an attack of optic neuritis is 50% in 15 years.[28] This can be stratified further, however, depending on lesion burden on baseline non–contrast-enhanced brain MRI. If a patient has a negative brain MRI at the time of diagnosis of optic neuritis, the risk of developing MS in the following 15 years is reduced to 25%. If 1 or more lesions are present on brain MRI, however, the risk increases to 72%. This information can be useful in counseling patients regarding their prognosis and need for serial monitoring. **Fig. 4** shows the brain MRI of the patient described in **Fig. 1**.

Long-term Therapy

Given the findings of the ONTT and the known risk of developing MS in the setting of optic neuritis, the Controlled High Risk Avonex Multiple Sclerosis Prevention Study (CHAMPS) evaluated the role of early disease-modifying therapy in reducing the rate of conversion to clinically definite MS.[29,30] Patients with optic neuritis or other acute demyelinating event and evidence of subclinical demyelination on brain MRI

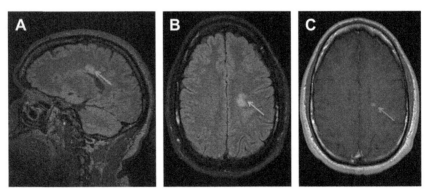

Fig. 4. Brain MRI of patient described in **Fig. 1.** (*A*) Sagittal T2 fluid-attenuated inversion recovery sequence image showing increased signal within the right posterior limb of the corpus callosum (*arrow*). (*B*) Axial fluid-attenuated inversion recovery sequence image showing increased signal in the left posterior frontal lobe (*arrow*), which enhances as seen in the axial postcontrast T1 image (*C*) (*arrow*).

were given IV corticosteroids and randomized to receive placebo or weekly intramuscular injections of interferon beta-1a (Avonex) and followed for 3 years. Interferon beta-1a was shown to reduce the development of clinically definite MS and the development of new brain lesions on MRI.

Similar to the CHAMPS study, the Early Treatment of Multiple Sclerosis (ETOMS) study showed a benefit from early interferon beta-1a treatment.[31] Patients were randomized to weekly interferon beta-1a (Rebif) or placebo after a first episode of demyelinating disease. Treated patients had a lower risk of developing MS in the first 2 years (34% vs 45% for placebo), a lower annual relapse rate (0.33 vs 0.43 for placebo), and a lower disease burden on MRI. Therefore, there is strong evidence of benefit for early treatment with disease-modifying therapies after an episode of optic neuritis in a high-risk population, defined by 2 or more lesions on brain MRI. **Table 1** summarizes the 3 landmark trials (discussed previously).

Subclinical Optic Neuritis

Some patients who never report symptoms consistent with an acute episode of optic neuritis may have findings on examination consistent with optic neuropathy, decreased acuity, reduced contrast sensitivity, dyschromatopsia, visual field defects, and optic atrophy.[32,33] rNFL atrophy on OCT can be seen in eyes of patients without

Table 1
Treatment after episode of acute optic neuritis

Trial	Medication	Outcomes
ONTT	Methylprednisolone	Faster recovery of visual function. Reduced rate of developing MS in first 2 y
CHAMPS	Interferon beta-1a	Reduced rate of developing MS in first 3 y Fewer new or enhancing lesions on MRI
ETOMS	Interferon beta-1a	Reduced rate of developing MS in first 2 y Fewer lesions on MRI Decreased annual relapse rate

prior episodes of optic neuritis and has been shown to correlate with lesion burden on brain MRI.[17,34,35] Serial monitoring of rNFL thickness on OCT in MS patients may be beneficial; however, further study in the area is needed.

NEUROMYELITIS OPTICA

NMO is an inflammatory autoimmune disease that preferentially attacks the optic nerves and spinal cord. Diagnostic criteria include a clinical history of both optic neuritis and transverse myelitis and at least 2 of 3 of the following supportive criteria: brain MRI not diagnostic of MS, spinal MRI with greater than or equal to 3 segment contiguous lesion, and aquaporin 4-IgG seropositivity.[20] The optic neuritis associated with NMO is often bilateral in onset, with more severe vision loss (<20/200) and more severe visual field depression.[36,37] Bilateral simultaneous optic neuritis, posterior optic nerve or chiasmal involvement, and poor visual recovery should prompt an evaluation for possible NMO. It is important to make the diagnosis of NMO early on because the prognosis for recovery is not as likely compared with optic neuritis in MS. In addition, the use of certain disease-modifying agents, such as beta interferons, natalizumab (Tysabri), and fingolimod (Gilenya), may actually worsen disease activity in NMO.[38–42]

OTHER AFFERENT VISUAL PATHWAY LESIONS

Chiasmal or retrochiasmal demyelination leading to bilateral visual field defects is less common in MS. In the ONTT, 5.1% of patients were found to have bitemporal visual field defects, consistent with chiasmal lesions, and 8.9% had homonymous hemianopias, seen in retrochiasmal disease.[7,43] The presence of chiasmal involvement in acute optic neuritis should prompt an investigation into possible NMO (discussed previously). Retrochiasmal lesions may occur anywhere along the posterior visual pathway, from the optic tracts to the optic radiations, with large lesions required to create significant visual field defects.[44] Patients with large homonymous or bitemporal visual field defects need to be counseled on whether they are safe to drive, the requirements for which vary by state. Additionally, homonymous hemianopias may make it difficult for a patient to read. Holding a straight edge along the line of text may be helpful. Some patients benefit from turning the text 90° vertically, with a left homonymous hemianopic patient reading up and a right homonymous hemianopic patient reading down, thereby always keeping the next line of text in the preserved visual field. Occasionally prism glasses are used to shift the visual field toward the affected side.

NYSTAGMUS

Nystagmus is a frequent finding in MS, observed in approximately 30% of patients.[45] Several different forms of nystagmus can be seen (listed in **Box 2**).[46–50] Nystagmus may be asymptomatic or cause oscillopsia, which can be variably bothersome depending on eye position.

The most common type of nystagmus associated with MS is gaze-evoked nystagmus, in which in eccentric gazes (typically in lateral and up gazes), the eyes beat away from the direction they are positioned.[45,51] This can cause oscillopsia when patients are looking away from primary position. Gaze evoked nystagmus is due to a lesion in the cerebellum or connection between the cerebellum and brainstem and can also be seen secondary to certain medications, such as anticonvulsants, sedatives, and antidepressants. Because the symptoms are not present in primary position, there is rarely an indication for treatment.

Box 2
Nystagmus in multiple sclerosis

Gaze-evoked nystagmus

Acquired pendular nystagmus

Torsional nystagmus

Upbeat or downbeat nystagmus

Abducting nystagmus associated with INO

Another common form of nystagmus in MS is acquired pendular nystagmus (APN).[52,53] In this type, the eyes move in a pendular fashion in the horizontal, vertical, and/or torsional planes. In addition to MS, APN can be seen in severe vision loss states, oculopalatal tremor, and spinocerebellar degeneration. The 2 eyes are often dissociated with variable amplitudes and frequencies. APN can be debilitating due to constant oscillopsia without a null point. Medications shown to be effective in dampening APN, including starting and maximum doses, are summarized in **Table 2**.[54–57]

Other defects in gaze holding, such as saccadic dysmetria and saccadic intrusions, are common in MS and usually seen in the setting of other eye movement abnormalities.[45,51] Lesions in the cerebellum can lead to hypometric or hypermetric saccades.[58] Square wave jerks, a type of saccadic intrusion, are rapid inappropriate movements away from and back to the target of fixation. Patients may report oscillopsia or difficulty with visual tasks. Saccadic intrusions may respond to baclofen or a variety of anticonvulsants.[2]

INTERNUCLEAR OPHTHALMOPLEGIA

Internuclear ophthalmoplegia (INO) is characterized by limited or slowed adduction in the affected eye, most easily observed during saccadic eye movements.[59] Often there is associated abducting nystagmus in the contralateral eye and spared convergence. An INO is caused by a lesion in the medial longitudinal fasciculus. Although an INO in an elderly patient is most commonly secondary to an ischemic stroke, the presence of an INO in a young otherwise healthy patient should prompt an evaluation for possible demyelinating disease.[60,61] The incidence of INO in MS patients is approximately 25%.[45] The findings of an INO may, however, be subtle on examination and can often be missed by an inexperienced examiner, so the diagnosis is likely greatly under-reported.[62] Patients may be asymptomatic, complain of diplopia or oscillopsia, or have vague eye tracking complaints.[63] Bilateral INO can occasionally manifest with

---

Table 2
Medications and dosages used to treat APN

Medication	Starting Dose (Oral Unless Specified)	Maximum Dose
Gabapentin	100 mg tid	1200 mg tid
Memantine	5 mg qd	10 mg bid
Clonazepam	0.5 mg tid	6.5 mg tid
Valproate	10 mg/kg/d in 1–3 Divided doses	60 mg/kg/d in 2–3 Divided doses
Scopolamine	1.5 mg Transdermal every 3 d	

a large angle exotropia (wall-eyed bilateral INO) causing diplopia and can be associated with vertical eye movement disorders, such as a skew deviation.[2] As with other demyelinating events, symptoms from INO may improve with time and with administration of IV steroids.[61] Occasionally, patients may require prism glasses or strabismus surgery to resolve their diplopia.

ONE-AND-A-HALF SYNDROME

One-and-a-half syndrome results from a lesion involving the abducens nucleus and/or the paramedian pontine reticular formation and the medial longitudinal fasciculus and manifests with an ipsilateral conjugate horizontal gaze palsy and associated ipsilateral adduction deficit.[64] Patients are left with the ability to abduct the contralateral eye only. Although typically seen in the setting of cerebral infarction, patients with MS may have a demyelinating lesion in the pons, leading to one-and-a-half syndrome. Symptoms can include diplopia and difficulty looking to the affected side.

CRANIAL NERVE PALSIES

Isolated 3rd, 4th, and 6th cranial nerve palsies, although rare in MS, should prompt an evaluation of demyelinating disease in otherwise young healthy patients who present with acute onset of diplopia.[65-69] Patients present with acute onset of binocular diplopia in a pattern consistent with the cranial nerve affected, with the sixth nerve the most commonly involved. Early management can include symptomatic occlusion and/or Fresnel lens placement. Occasionally, patients require strabismus surgery to realign the eyes and resolve the diplopia in stable palsies; however, more typically there is complete spontaneous recovery over a period of weeks. There is no proved benefit of eye muscle exercises in the treatment of cranial nerve palsies.

OTHER EFFERENT VISUAL PATHWAY LESIONS

A skew deviation is a vertical misalignment of the eyes, caused by a lesion in the pathways connecting the vestibular nuclei in the medulla with the 3rd and 4th cranial nerve nuclei in the midbrain.[70] The pattern of the deviation typically does not map out in a pattern consistent with a cranial nerve palsy. Patients may complain of binocular vertical diplopia. As with other causes of diplopia, occlusion or Fresnel lenses may help, and, rarely, patients require surgical intervention.

Dorsal midbrain, or Parinaud, syndrome is a group of findings, including a supranuclear upgaze palsy, convergence-retraction nystagmus, eyelid retraction, and light-near dissociation secondary to a lesion in the posterior midbrain.[71] Although the most common cause in a young patient is a pineal tumor, demyelinating disease is a well-known cause of this syndrome.[72,73] Infrequently, patients with significant upgaze paresis may require bilateral inferior rectus recessions to shift the eyes into primary position.[74]

UVEITIS

Intraocular inflammation, including anterior uveitis, pars planitis, and retinal phlebitis, is a rare manifestation of MS, with an incidence of approximately 1%; however, this is 10-fold higher than in the general population.[75-77] A diagnosis of uveitis may precede or follow a diagnosis of MS.[78] The most common uveitic presentation in MS patients is intermediate uveitis or pars planitis characterized by intravitreal inflammation, with pars plana exudates and snowbanking, most typically with bilateral disease.[79,80] Patients may be asymptomatic or complain of floaters and/or blurred vision. Other

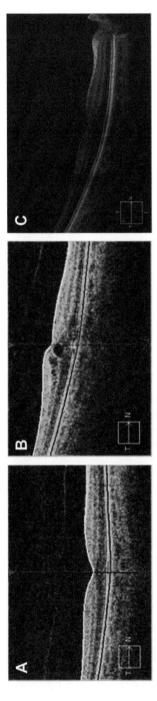

Fig. 5. Spectral domain OCT scans of a patient who developed macular edema while taking fingolimod. (A) Baseline macular OCT prior to starting fingolimod, showing normal retinal architecture and foveal depression in the right eye. (B) Shows the development of macular edema right eye, 4 weeks after starting fingolimod. After discontinuing fingolimod, the macular edema resolved (C). (*Courtesy of* Steven R. Hamilton, MD, Neuro-ophthalmic Consultants Northwest, Seattle, Washington.)

infectious or autoimmune causes, such as syphilis, tuberculosis, and sarcoidosis, must be considered. Studies have reported a range of 33% to 47.6% of patients with pars planitis having concurrent MS.[80,81] Therefore, most patients found to have pars planitis, and certainly those with a positive neurologic review of systems, should undergo neuroimaging. Pars planitis is treated with topical, local, or systemic steroids, nonsteroidal agents, and other systemic immunosuppressants. Complications include macular edema, epiretinal membrane formation, and cataracts.

Rarely, patients with MS may develop anterior uveitis and present with pain, photophobia, and decreased vision in 1 or both eyes. The inflammation may be granulomatous or nongranulomatous and other infectious or inflammatory etiologies must be considered, including syphilis, tuberculosis, sarcoidosis, and other rheumatologic disorders. Complications include cataract, glaucoma, and macular edema. Anterior uveitis is typically treated with topical and/or local corticosteroids and topical cycloplegics.

COMPLICATIONS OF TREATMENT OF MULTIPLE SCLEROSIS

Fingolimod became the first oral drug Food and Drug Administration approved for the treatment of MS in 2010. It is a sphingosine 1-phosphate receptor analog, which causes internalization and down-regulation of sphingosine 1-phosphate receptors, thereby preventing the release of lymphocytes from lymph nodes.[82] Two large phase 3 clinical trials, FREEDOMS (FTY720 Research Evaluating Effects of Daily Oral therapy in Multiple Sclerosis) and TRANSFORMS (Trial Assessing Injectable Interferon versus FTY720 Oral in Relapsing—Remitting Multiple Sclerosis), showed decreased rates of relapse compared with placebo or weekly intramuscular interferon beta-1a, respectively.[83,84] In the TRANSFORMS trial, 2 patients (0.5%) given fingolimod (0.5 mg daily) developed macular edema. Macular edema may be asymptomatic but can lead to decreased vision or metamorphopsia (distortion of vision). The package insert for fingolimod reports the incidence of macular edema to be 0.4%.[85] In patients with a history of diabetes or uveitis, the risk of macular edema greatly increases to up to 20%. Because the incidence of uveitis in MS patients is significantly higher than in the general population, it is important to screen patients for previously undiagnosed intraocular inflammation.

Given the association between fingolimod and macular edema, all patients considered for fingolimod therapy are advised to have a dilated fundus examination prior to starting the medication and a repeat examination 3 to 4 months after being on the medication, sooner if any changes in vision develop.[86] If macular edema develops, drug cessation should be considered. The use of macular OCT may be helpful in the evaluation of patients with visual complaints when taking fingolimod. **Fig. 5** shows an OCT of patient who developed macular edema when taking fingolimod. The edema resolved after cessation of therapy.

Progressive multifocal leukoencephalopathy (PML) has been linked to natalizumab therapy in patients exposed to the JC virus, in particular those with a high number of infusions.[87] PML may present with several neurologic manifestations, including visual impairment.[88] A recent review noted 29% of patients with natalizumab-associated PML presented with visual impairment, with a majority of those patients having a homonymous hemianopia.[87] The development of a new homonymous hemianopia in a patient with a history of natalizumab therapy should prompt an evaluation for possible PML.

SUMMARY

As discussed previously, MS can have many manifestations that affect a patient's vision. Optic neuritis is common and typically has a good outcome. Many patients are left with some residual deficits, however, such as reduced contrast sensitivity. rNFL OCT can document the progression of optic atrophy in the setting of optic neuritis and additionally can be used as a likely biomarker for disease activity in MS. Efferent visual pathway disorders, including nystagmus, INO, and saccadic dysfunction, are likely greatly underappreciated and may add to a patient's visual impairment. The association between MS and uveitis is important to remember because more patients are started on fingolimod therapy. An awareness of the many potential visual symptoms in MS is important in managing patients and maximizing their vision and quality of life.

REFERENCES

1. Jacobs DA, Galetta SL. Multiple sclerosis and the visual system. Ophthalmol Clin North Am 2004;17:265–73.
2. Frohman EM, Frohman TC, Zee DS, et al. The neuro-ophthalmology of multiple sclerosis. Lancet Neurol 2005;4:111–21.
3. Foroozan R, Buono LM, Savino PJ, et al. Acute demyelinating optic neuritis. Curr Opin Ophthalmol 2002;13:375–80.
4. Miller D, Barkhof F, Montalban X, et al. Clinically isolated syndromes suggestive of multiple sclerosis, part 1: natural history, pathogenesis, diagnosis, and prognosis. Lancet Neurol 2005;4:281–8.
5. Agostini E, Frigerio R, Protti A. Controversies in optic neuritis pain diagnosis. Neurol Sci 2005;26(Suppl 2):s75–8.
6. The clinical profile of optic neuritis: experience of the Optic Neuritis Treatment Trial. Optic Neuritis Study Group. Arch Ophthalmol 1991;109:1673–8.
7. Keltner JL, Johnson CA, Spurr JO, et al. Baseline visual field profile of optic neuritis: the experience of the Optic Neuritis Treatment Trial. Optic Neuritis Study Group. Arch Ophthalmol 1993;111:231–4.
8. Beck RW, Trobe JD, Moke PS, et al. High- and low-risk profiles for the development of multiple sclerosis within 10 years after optic neuritis: experience of the Optic Neuritis Treatment Trial. Arch Ophthalmol 2003;121:944–9.
9. The 5-year risk of MS after optic neuritis. Experience of the Optic Neuritis Treatment Trial. Optic Neuritis Treatment Group. Neurology 1997;49:1404–13.
10. Eggenberger E. Inflammatory optic neuropathies. Ophthalmol Clin North Am 2001;14:73–82.
11. Rizzo JF, Andreoli CM, Rabinov JD. Use of magnetic resonance imaging to differentiate optic neuritis and nonarteritic anterior ischemic optic neuropathy. Ophthalmology 2002;109:1679–84.
12. Hickman SJ, Miszkiel KA, Plant GT, et al. The optic nerve sheath on MRI in acute optic neuritis. Neuroradiology 2005;47:51–5.
13. Hickman SJ. Optic nerve imaging in multiple sclerosis. J Neuroimaging 2007; 17(Suppl 1):S42–5.
14. Costello F, Coupland S, Hodge W, et al. Quantifying axonal loss after optic neuritis with optical coherence tomography. Ann Neurol 2006;59:963–9.
15. Costello F, Hodge W, Pan YI, et al. Tracking retinal nerve fiber layer loss after optic neuritis: a prospective study using optic coherence tomography. Mult Scler 2008;14:898–905.
16. Trip SA, Schlottmann PG, Jones SJ, et al. Retinal nerve fiber layer axonal loss and visual dysfunction in optic neuritis. Ann Neurol 2005;58:383–91.
17. Gordon-Lipkin E, Chodkowski B, Reich DS, et al. Retinal nerve fiber layer is associated with brain atrophy in multiple sclerosis. Neurology 2007;69:1603–9.

18. Optic nerve decompression surgery for nonarteritic anterior ischemic optic neuropathy (NAION) is not effective and may be harmful. The Ischemic Optic Neuropathy Decompression Trial Research Group. JAMA 1995;273:625–32.

19. Hickman SJ, Dalton CM, Miller DH, et al. Management of acute optic neuritis. Lancet 2002;360:1953–62.

20. Wingerchuk DM, Lennon VA, Pittock SJ, et al. Revised diagnostic criteria for neuromyelitis optica. Neurology 2006;66:1485–9.

21. Beck RW. The Optic Neuritis Treatment Trial. Arch Ophthalmol 1988;106: 1051–3.

22. Beck RW, Cleary PA, Anderson MM, et al. The Optic Neuritis Study Group. A randomized, controlled trial of corticosteroids in the treatment of optic neuritis. N Engl J Med 1992;326:581–8.

23. Beck RW, Cleary PA. Optic Neuritis Treatment Trial. One-year follow-up results. Arch Ophthalmol 1993;111:773–5.

24. Beck RW. The Optic Neuritis Treatment Trial: three-year follow-up results. Arch Ophthalmol 1995;113:136–7.

25. Beck RW, Gal RL, Bhatti MT, et al. Visual function more than 10 years after optic neuritis: experience of the Optic Neuritis Treatment Trial. Am J Ophthalmol 2004; 137:77–83.

26. Beck RW, Cleary PA, Trobe JD, et al. The effect of corticosteroids for acute optic neuritis on the subsequent development of multiple sclerosis. N Engl J Med 1993;329:1764–9.

27. Optic Neuritis Study Group. Visual function 15 years after optic neuritis: A final follow-up report from the Optic Neuritis Treatment Trial. Ophthalmology 2008; 115:1079–82.

28. The Optic Neuritis Study Group. Multiple sclerosis risk after optic neuritis: Final Optic Neuritis Treatment Trial follow-up. Arch Neurol 2008;65:727–32.

29. Jacobs LD, Beck RW, Simon JH, et al. Intramuscular interferon beta-1a therapy initiated during a first demyelinating event in multiple sclerosis. N Engl J Med 2000;343:898–904.

30. CHAMPS Study Group. Interferon ß-1a for optic neuritis patients at high risk for multiple sclerosis. Am J Ophthalmol 2001;132:463–71.

31. Comi G, Filippi M, Barkhoff F, et al. Effect of early interferon treatment on conversion to definite multiple sclerosis: a randomised study. Lancet 2001;357: 1576–82.

32. Baier ML, Cutter GR, Rudick RA, et al. Low-contrast letter acuity testing captures visual dysfunction in patients with multiple sclerosis. Neurology 2005;64: 992–5.

33. Zaveri MS, Conger A, Salter A, et al. Retinal imaging by laser polarimetry and optical coherence tomography evidence of axonal degeneration in multiple sclerosis. Arch Neurol 2008;65:924–8.

34. Siger M, Dziegielewski K, Jasek L, et al. Optical coherence tomography in multiple sclerosis: thickness of the retinal nerve fiber layer as a potential measure of axonal loss and brain atrophy. J Neurol 2008;255:1555–60.

35. Grazioli E, Zivadinov R, Weinstock-Guttman B, et al. Retinal nerve fiber layer thickness is associated with brain MRI outcomes in multiple sclerosis. J Neurol Sci 2008;268:12–7.

36. Merle H, Olindo S, Bonnan M, et al. Natural history of the visual impairment of relapsing neuromyelitis optica. Ophthalmology 2007;114:810–5.

37. Wingerchuk DM, Hogancamp WF, O'Brien PC, et al. The clinical course of neuromyelitis optica (Devic's syndrome). Neurology 1999;53:1107–14.

38. Palace J, Leite MI, Nairne A, et al. Interferon beta treatment in neuromyelitis optica: increase in relapses and aquaporin 4 antibody titers. Arch Neurol 2010;67:1016–7.

39. Papeix C, Vidal JS, de Seze J, et al. Immunosuppressive therapy is more effective than interferon in neuromyelitis optica. Mult Scler 2007;13:256–9.

40. Shimizu J, Hatanaka Y, Hasegawa M, et al. IFNß-1b may severely exacerbate Japanese optic-spinal MS in neuromyelitis optica spectrum. Neurology 2010; 75:1423–7.

41. Kleiter I, Hellwig K, Berthele A, et al. Failure of natalizumab to prevent relapses in neuromyelitis optica. Arch Neurol 2012;69:239–45.

42. Min JH, Kim BJ, Lee KH. Development of extensive brain lesions following fingolimod (FTY720) treatment in a patient with neuromyelitis optica spectrum disorder. Mult Scler 2012;18:113–5.

43. Keltner JL, Johnson CA, Spurr JO, et al. Visual field profile of optic neuritis. One-year follow-up in the Optic Neuritis Treatment Trial. Arch Ophthalmol 1994;112:946–53.

44. Plant GT, Kermode AG, Turano G, et al. Symptomatic retrochiasmal lesions in multiple sclerosis: clinical features, visual evoked potentials, and magnetic resonance imaging. Neurology 1992;42:68–76.

45. Serra A, Derwenskus J, Downey DL, et al. Role of eye movement examination and subjective visual vertical in clinical evaluation of multiple sclerosis. J Neurol 2003;250:569–75.

46. Sandramouli S, Benamer HT, Mantle M, et al. See-saw nystagmus as the presenting sign in multiple sclerosis. J Neuroophthalmol 2005;25:56–7.

47. Matsumoto S, Ohyagi Y, Inoue I, et al. Periodic alternating nystagmus in a patient with MS. Neurology 2001;56:276–7.

48. Keane JR. Periodic alternating nystagmus with downward beating nystagmus. A clinicoanatomical case study of multiple sclerosis. Arch Neurol 1974;30: 399–402.

49. Halmagyi GM, Aw ST, Dehaene I, et al. Jerk-waveform see-saw nystagmus due to unilateral meso-diencephalic lesion. Brain 1994;117(Pt 4):789–803.

50. Ohkoshi N, Komatsu Y, Mizusawa H, et al. Primary position upbeat nystagmus increased on downward gaze: clinicopathologic study of a patient with multiple sclerosis. Neurology 1998;50:551–3.

51. Downey DL, Stahl JS, Bhidayasiri R, et al. Saccadic and vestibular abnormalities in multiple sclerosis: sensitive clinical signs of brainstem and cerebellar involvement. Ann N Y Acad Sci 2002;956:438–40.

52. Averbuch-Heller L, Zivotofsky AZ, Das VE, et al. Investigations of the pathogenesis of acquired pendular nystagmus. Brain 1995;118(Pt 2):369–78.

53. Barton JJ, Cox TA. Acquired pendular nystagmus in multiple sclerosis: clinical observations and the role of optic neuropathy. J Neurol Neurosurg Psychiatry 1993;56:262–7.

54. Averbuch-Heller L, Tusa RJ, Fuhry L, et al. A double-blind controlled study of gabapentin and baclofen as treatment for acquired nystagmus. Ann Neurol 1997;41:818–25.

55. Starck M, Albrecht H, Pollman W, et al. Drug therapy for acquired pendular nystagmus in multiple sclerosis. J Neurol 1997;244:9–16.

56. Rucker JC. Current treatment of nystagmus. Curr Treat Options Neurol 2005;7: 69–77.

57. Leigh RJ, Tomsak RL. Drug treatments for eye movement disorders. J Neurol Neurosurg Psychiatry 2003;74:1–4.

58. Lewis RF, Zee DS. Ocular motor disorders associated with cerebellar lesions: pathophysiology and topical localization. Rev Neurol (Paris) 1993;149:665–77.
59. Zee DS. Internuclear ophthalmoplegia: pathophysiology and diagnosis. Baillieres Clin Neurol 1992;1:455–70.
60. Keane JR. Internuclear ophthalmoplegia: unusual causes in 114 of 410 patients. Arch Neurol 2005;62:714–7.
61. Bolanos I, Lozano D, Cantu C. Internuclear ophthalmoplegia: causes and long-term follow-up in 65 patients. Acta Neurol Scand 2004;110:161–5.
62. Frohman TC, Frohman EM, O'Suilleabhain P, et al. Accuracy of clinical detection of INO in MS: corroboration with quantitative infrared oculography. Neurology 2003;61:848–50.
63. Mills DA, Frohman TC, Davis SL, et al. Break in fusion during head turning in MS patients with INO. Neurology 2008;71:458–60.
64. Wall M, Wray SH. The one-and-a-half syndrome – a unilateral disorder of the pontine tegmentum: a study of 20 cases and review of the literature. Neurology 1983;33:971–80.
65. Thomke F, Lensch E, Ringel K, et al. Isolated cranial nerve palsies in multiple sclerosis. J Neurol Neurosurg Psychiatry 1997;63:682–5.
66. Zadro I, Barun B, Habek M, et al. Isolated cranial nerve palsies in multiple sclerosis. Clin Neurol Neurosurg 2008;110:886–8.
67. Bentley PI, Kimber T, Schapira AH. Painful third nerve palsy in MS. Neurology 2002;58:1532.
68. Jacobson DM, Moster ML, Eggenberger ER, et al. Isolated trochlear nerve palsy in patients with multiple sclerosis. Neurology 1999;53:877–9.
69. Moster ML, Savino PL, Sergott RC, et al. Isolated sixth-nerve palsies in younger adults. Arch Ophthalmol 1984;102:1328–30.
70. Brodsky MC, Donahue SP, Vaphiades M, et al. Skew deviation revisited. Surv Ophthalmol 2006;51:105–28.
71. Parinaud H. Paralysie des mouvements associés des yeux. Archives de neurologie, Paris 1883;5:145–72.
72. Frohman EM, Dewey RB, Frohman TC. An unsual variant of the dorsal midbrain syndrome in MS: clinical characteristics and pathophysiologic mechanisms. Mult Scler 2004;10:322–5.
73. Lee WB, Berger JR, O'Halloran HS. Parinaud syndrome heralding MS. Neurology 2003;60:322.
74. Buckley EG, Holgado S. Surgical treatment of upgaze palsy in Parinaud's syndrome. J AAPOS 2004;8:249–53.
75. Smith JR, Rosenbaum JT. Neurological concomitants of uveitis. Br J Ophthalmol 2004;88:1498–9.
76. Biousse V, Trichet C, Bloch-Michel E, et al. Multiple sclerosis associated with uveitis in two large clinic-based series. Neurology 1999;52:179–81.
77. Chen L, Gordon LK. Ocular manifestations of multiple sclerosis. Curr Opin Ophthalmol 2005;16:315–20.
78. Zein G, Berta A, Foster CS. Mulitple sclerosis-associated uveitis. Ocul Immunol Inflamm 2004;12:137–42.
79. Towler HM, Lightman S. Symptomatic intraocular inflammation in multiple sclerosis. Clin Experiment Ophthalmol 2000;28:97–102.
80. Raja SC, Jabs DA, Dunn JP, et al. Pars planitis: clinical features and class II HLA associations. Ophthalmology 1999;106:594–9.
81. Prieto JF, Dios E, Gutierrez JM, et al. Pars planitis: epidemiology, treatment and association with multiple sclerosis. Ocul Immunol Inflamm 2001;9:93–102.

82. Mandala S, Hajdu R, Bergstrom J, et al. Alteration of lymphocyte trafficking by sphingosine-1-phosphate receptor agonists. Science 2002;296:346–9.

83. Kappos L, Radue EW, O'Connor P, et al. A placebo-controlled trial of oral fingolimod in relapsing multiple sclerosis. N Engl J Med 2010;362:387–401.

84. Cohen JA, Barkhof F, Comi G, et al. Oral fingolimod or intramuscular interferon for relapsing multiple sclerosis. N Engl J Med 2010;362:402–15.

85. Highlights of prescribing information: Gilenya (fingolimod) capsules. Novartis; 2012.

86. Lee AG, Ophthalmic News & Education (ONE) Network Neuro-Ophthalmology Committee, Oral MS drug may increase risk for macular edema: a report from the North American Neuro-Ophthalmology Society (NANOS) and the AAO, ONE Network Neuro-Ophthalmology Committee; 2011.

87. Clifford DB, DeLuca A, Simpson DM, et al. Natalizumab-associated progressive multifocal leukoencephalopathy in patients with multiple sclerosis: lessons from 28 cases. Lancet Neurol 2010;9:438–46.

88. Brooks BR, Walker DL. Progressive multifocal leukoencephalopathy. Neurol Clin 1984;2:299–313.

Co-occurring Depression and Pain in Multiple Sclerosis

Kevin N. Alschuler, PhD*, Dawn M. Ehde, PhD, Mark P. Jensen, PhD

KEYWORDS

- Depression • Pain • Multiple sclerosis

KEY POINTS

- Depression and pain are highly prevalent among individuals with multiple sclerosis (MS), often co-occur, and likely make each other worse.
- Both depression and pain impact quality of life, medical utilization, and the effectiveness of interventions.
- Although there are effective interventions for depression and pain, no interventions have yet been developed that target comorbid pain and depression in individuals with MS.

INTRODUCTION

A classic element of multiple sclerosis (MS) is the presence of multiple symptoms that impact functioning. In prior reviews,[1,2] the authors have commented on the significance of individual problems, specifically pain and depression, reporting on prevalence rates and outlining recommendations for the treatment of each one individually. The reality, however, is that these problems often co-occur and likely have bidirectional effects, with each amplifying the other. The purpose of this article is to summarize the theory and existing literature on the comorbidity of pain and depression and describe how their presence impacts individuals with MS. Additionally, the article discusses how existing treatments for pain and depression could be adapted to address shared mechanisms and overcome barriers to treatment utilization.

Sources of support: The contents of this article were developed under grants from: (1) the Institutes of Health, National Institute of Child Health and Human Development, National Center for Medical Rehabilitation Research (grant number R01HD057916); (2) the National Multiple Sclerosis Society (grant number MB 0008); and (3) the Department of Education (grant number H133B080025). The article does not necessarily represent the policy of the Department of Education, and you should not assume endorsement by the federal government.
Department of Rehabilitation Medicine, University of Washington School of Medicine, Box 358815, 1536 North 115th Street, Seattle, WA 98133, USA
* Corresponding author. Department of Rehabilitation Medicine, UW Medicine Multiple Sclerosis Center, University of Washington School of Medicine, Box 358815, 1536 North 115th Street, Seattle, WA 98133.
E-mail address: kalschul@uw.edu

PREVALENCE OF PAIN, DEPRESSION, AND THEIR COMORBIDITY

Several prior studies have reported that pain and depression are both common in individuals with MS. For example, 50% of the people with MS in clinical samples are reported to experience chronic pain at any one point in time.[3] In a community sample of people with MS and pain, 75% reported experiencing some pain and 40% reported an average pain severity of 3 or greater on a scale of 0 to 10,[4] which is understood to be pain of at least moderate intensity in people with MS.[5] In another community sample of people with MS and pain, 25% described their pain as severe.[6]

The 12-month prevalence of major depressive disorder in people with MS is about twice that of the general population (15.7% vs 7.4%, respectively).[7] The lifetime prevalence of depressive disorders in MS is 2 to 3 times that of the general population.[2,8] Many people with MS, as high as 50% at any one time, experience depressive symptoms that may not always reflect a clinical diagnosis of a mood disorder but are nonetheless clinically significant.[9–12]

Although many studies described the associations between pain and depressive symptoms in individuals with MS, few have reported on the prevalence of their co-occurrence.[3,6,13,14] A recent study using varying criteria to identify depression and pain in a community sample of people with MS reported that pain and depression co-occurred in 6% to 19% of the sample, depending on which criteria for pain and depression were used.[4] Pain was experienced by 86% to 100% of people meeting depression criteria, and pain of moderate severity was experienced by 67% to 77% of people meeting depression criteria. In contrast, 11% to 34% of people experiencing *any* pain met depression criteria and 15% to 37% of people experiencing pain of at least moderate severity met criteria for clinical depression. In a prior study of a community sample of people with MS, 53% of the people with pain reported having clinically significant levels of depressive symptoms.[6]

AMPLIFYING EFFECTS OF PAIN AND DEPRESSION ON ONE ANOTHER

Prior MS research has reported high associations between pain and depression, such that higher pain is associated with worse depressive symptoms.[3,6,13,14] This finding suggests the possibility that the presence of one condition amplifies the presence or severity of the other. Indeed, cross-sectional studies in MS[4] and longitudinal studies in the general population[15–17] have shown that chronic pain is a risk factor for subsequent depression; similarly, depression is a risk factor for chronic pain. At the same time, a substantial percentage of individuals with MS have only pain or depression,[4] suggesting that there may be both overlapping and unique aspects of the two conditions.[16]

When looking at studies in this area in individuals who do not have MS, the evidence is mixed regarding whether pain has a larger impact on depression than depression has on pain. For example, an earlier review of 191 studies examining the association between pain and depression in a large variety of patient and nonpatient samples reported consistent support for the *consequence* hypothesis (depression is influenced by the presence or severity of chronic pain) and inconsistent support for the *antecedent* hypothesis (depression precedes pain).[18] A recent longitudinal study of 95 adolescents diagnosed with chronic pain or depression reported evidence for a bidirectional association between depression and pain, although the impact of pain on depression was stronger than the impact of depression on pain.[19] In contrast, a study of 500 primary care patients with chronic musculoskeletal pain demonstrated that the two had an equally adverse impact on the other.[16] In their sample, change in severity of either depression or pain predicted a change in severity of the other symptom over time. Longitudinal research tracking pain and depression in people with MS would illuminate the nature and consequences of their relationships over time.

In the research literature outside of MS, researchers have suggested several reasons why pain and depression co-occur and why the presence of either pain or depression makes the other more likely.[15,16,18] In terms of pathophysiology, prior reviews of depression and pain have noted that central nociceptive and affective pathways overlap,[15,18] which supports the understanding that chronic pain is modulated centrally.[20] The experience of depressive symptoms and pain also share underlying neurotransmitters, with both norepinephrine and serotonin implicated in mood disorders and in the processing of pain. Beyond pathophysiology, there are potential psychological and behavioral reasons that pain and depression may amplify one another. For example, depressive symptoms have been found to impact the evaluative and affective aspects of pain and pain-related disability.[21,22] Pain often impacts the extent to which individuals engage in physical activity, which can limit an individual's participation in activities that were previously valued or enjoyed and, thus, puts the individual at risk for low mood.[23] Although it is highly likely that these same mechanisms play a role in individuals with MS, additional research is needed to understand the importance of these mechanisms and to understand whether additional, unique factors may also be implicated in the MS population.

OVERLAPPING IMPACT OF PAIN AND DEPRESSION ON FUNCTIONING AND QUALITY OF LIFE

Depression and chronic pain have a significant negative impact on individuals living with MS.[24] Major depression is associated with poorer neuropsychological functioning, lower quality of life, increased time lost from work, social disruption, and poorer health. Chronic pain in MS has been associated with poorer health-related quality of life, including greater interference with daily activities, energy/vitality, mental health, and social functioning.[3,6] Depression and pain have been linked to higher risk for unemployment[25]; both are also thought to affect fatigue negatively, another common and often disabling symptom of MS. For example, people with MS and clinically significant depressive symptoms are 6.2 times more likely to have disabling fatigue than nondepressed controls with MS.[26] Studies in MS have highlighted that higher levels of depressive symptoms and pain are associated with lower quality of life independent of other confounding symptoms.[27–31] Furthermore, research in other medical populations has shown that pain and depression have a reciprocal and additive adverse impact on quality of life and disability.[16,32]

Depression and pain may also impact the ability of a person with MS to self-manage their condition and its effects on daily life. Depression is thought to affect self-management through its adverse effects on energy, motivation, concentration, self-efficacy, and interpersonal interactions.[33] For example, a meta-analysis found that people with depression and chronic medical illness had a 3-fold higher rate of nonadherence to self-care regimens compared with nondepressed controls.[34] Consistent with these findings, depression has been associated with a decreased ability to manage MS symptoms, including adherence to disease-modifying medications.[35–37] Individuals with MS and chronic pain are also more likely to be inactive[13] and to report lower self-efficacy for managing their MS, including pain.[38] The extent to which co-morbid pain and depression conjointly influence individuals' MS self-management is an area worthy of further exploration.

IMPACT ON TREATMENT UTILIZATION AND EFFECTIVENESS

Depression and pain likely influence health care utilization and treatment effectiveness. For example, in a recent study, the authors described how the rates of pain treatment utilization of patients with MS were higher among the subset of patients who were also depressed.[39] Individuals with comorbid pain and depression were found to have made more visits to medical providers for pain intervention, tried more pain treatments, and trended toward making more emergency department visits for pain intervention relative to individuals with pain alone. This finding is consistent with research in other medical populations that has shown that pain and depression are associated with higher rates of health care utilization.[40,41] In other medical conditions, pain and depression are also thought to reduce the effectiveness of treatments for the other condition (see Bair and colleagues[15,42] for a review of this literature). In other words, the presence of pain may interfere with depression treatment and vice versa. Such relationships have not been studied in people with MS, pain, and depression, however. Further, this prior research has suggested that the presence of pain distracts providers from detecting the presence of depression and subsequently results in the undertreatment of depression in pain populations.[15] Whether pain is a contributing factor to the underidentification and treatment of depression among patients with MS[11,43] is unknown.

INTERVENTIONS FOR COMORBID PAIN AND DEPRESSION

Descriptions of pharmacologic and cognitive-behavioral interventions for depression[2] and pain[1] have been provided in prior articles. However, the authors are unaware of research on combined treatments for depression and pain in MS, despite their co-occurrence and presumed bidirectional impact on each other. Effective treatment of depression has been shown to have a secondary effect of improving pain in primary care patients.[42] Research in other medical populations also points to the potential for successful treatment of comorbid pain and depression through antidepressant therapy, cognitive-behavioral therapy (CBT), and self-hypnosis training, although results have been far from definitive to this point.[15]

Antidepressants are commonly prescribed to patients with MS with neuropathic pain to address not only pain but also depression and sleep. However, little is known about the efficacy of antidepressants for treating neuropathic pain in MS.[13] Tricyclic antidepressants have some evidence for their efficacy in treating chronic pain in other neuropathic pain disorders,[44] although they are typically prescribed at doses lower than those needed for depression treatment. Side effects of tricyclic antidepressants can also be a deterrent to their use for pain and depression. There is also evidence that the serotonin-norepinephrine reuptake inhibitors duloxetine and venlafaxine are effective in the treatment of neuropathic pain in a range of conditions, although their efficacy in MS pain has not been studied.[13] Only a few antidepressants have been evaluated for their benefits in treating depression in MS via randomized controlled trials for depression,[45,46] and no studies were found reporting the benefits of treating depression with antidepressants on pain.

Among the available psychological treatments for depression and pain, CBT has the most evidence supporting its efficacy in individuals with MS. In a series of randomized controlled trials, Mohr and colleagues[35,46–49] demonstrated that CBT, delivered both in person and by telephone, is efficacious in reducing depression as well as fatigue, disability, and quality of life.[50] CBT for chronic pain has been less extensively studied in MS populations, although preliminary evidence in MS[51] and a substantial body of evidence in other painful conditions[52] support its use for chronic pain in MS. However, although CBT for depression and pain share many ingredients (such as relaxation training, cognitive restructuring, behavioral activation), treatments targeting both have not been developed or tested, to the authors' knowledge.

One of the treatments for pain with the longest history, hypnosis, had not been tested in controlled trials until recently. However, research has established its efficacy for several chronic pain conditions.[53,54] Even more recently, controlled trials of hypnosis in individuals with MS and chronic pain have demonstrated its efficacy for reducing pain intensity and pain interference.[55,56] In addition, preliminary research suggests that hypnotic interventions may also be effective for reducing depressive symptoms.[57–59] Although research is needed to confirm that hypnosis and hypnotic interventions are as effective in individuals with MS and depression as they are in individuals who present with pain or depression as a primary problem, there is no a priori reason to hypothesize the benefits would not generalize to an MS population.

UTILIZATION OF AND ACCESS TO INTERVENTIONS FOR COMORBID PAIN AND DEPRESSION

Outside of the development of treatments targeting the pain-depression comorbidity, a pressing issue is the ability of patients to access and appropriately use the interventions that are currently available. Specifically, prior research has shown that although effective treatments for pain and depression are available, these two conditions remain underidentified and undertreated in MS populations.[3,6,43,60] An estimated two-thirds of people with MS and major depression are untreated.[35,61,62] Similarly, although psychosocial interventions specifically targeting MS and depression have been found to be effective,[35] both real and perceived barriers impact the follow-through with depression treatment referrals.[63] The MS literature also reflects poor utilization of screening information to improve treatment referrals, even when screening is systematically implemented.[11] Pain is also inadequately treated; treatments that patients identify as most helpful are not necessarily the most frequently used, and nonpharmacologic pain management strategies are used at very low rates despite their potential to reduce pain and associated suffering.[55] (Ehde DM, Osborne TL, Hanley MA, et al. Use and perceived effectiveness of treatments for pain associated with multiple sclerosis. submitted for publication) These studies highlight the need to implement and evaluate new systems of care for pain and depression to address the undertreatment of depression and pain in people with MS.

INNOVATIVE APPROACHES TO THE MANAGEMENT OF COMORBID DEPRESSION AND PAIN

In other medical populations whereby depression and/or chronic pain are common, the collaborative care model has been found to be an effective systems-based approach to managing chronic comorbid conditions. This model emphasizes implementing systemic changes complete with self-management support, clinical information systems, delivery system redesign, decision support, health care organization, and community resources.[64,65] Health professionals are not simply colocated; they use established principles of chronic care management and interdisciplinary collaborative care teams in which professionals with complementary skills work closely together to care for a population of patients with complex medical conditions. Specialists and primary medical providers actively collaborate in providing integrated care, usually assisted by a care manager who guides patients collaboratively through various decisions about and aspects of care. The specialists, such as psychiatrists or pain specialists, supervise the care managers. The specialists are also available to consult primary medical providers on patients who are clinically challenging or who need additional specialty services and to see patients themselves when required. Collaborative care also typically features a stepped-care approach in which interventions are titrated based on the response to treatment. Collaborative care emphasizes measurement-based care, including screening and ongoing measurement and monitoring of treatment outcomes. Thus, the severity of problems such as depression and pain are repeatedly measured, and the treatment is systematically intensified or modified to ensure that the targeted improvements are achieved.

Collaborative care has repeatedly proven to be an effective model for maximizing access to, and efficacy of, medical treatment of chronic conditions. Collaborative care has improved depression outcomes and quality of care in patients with co-occurring chronic conditions, such as diabetes, coronary heart disease, and osteoarthritis.[60,66–72] A meta-analysis of 37 randomized controlled trials showed that collaborative care is more effective than standard care in improving short-term and long-term (up to 5 years) depression outcomes in primary care settings.[67] Recent trials have successfully tested collaborative care for patients with chronic pain (with or without depression) and produced useful benefits over usual care in improving pain, depression, and functional outcomes.[60,73–77]

The collaborative care approach is consistent with many of the conclusions of a 2002 MS stakeholder consensus conference on the identification and treatment of depression in MS.[43] Their recommendations for improving depression care in patients with MS included standardization of depression treatment, individualized care based on patient preferences, treatment to remission, and integrated biopsychosocial treatments that include options for both pharmacologic and psychosocial care.[43] Although they did not mention collaborative care in their published statement, their recommendations are consistent with a collaborative care model of depression care. Despite these recommendations made 10 years ago, collaborative care is not yet standard practice in MS care. In fact, the authors are aware of only one small, nonrandomized study that used the collaborative care model to treat depression in MS.[78] Results showed that at 6 months after baseline, fewer (33.3%) patients who received care management met diagnostic criteria for major depression relative to historical controls who received standard care (55.2%, $P = .15$). Although preliminary, this study supports the need for further evaluation of a collaborative care intervention, including by tailoring the intervention to match the needs of people with MS.

Given the tremendous barriers to receiving adequate behavioral health services,[79] an additional direction for future intervention development and research is the use of technology to deliver pain and depression care. Although not previously studied in people with MS, literature from other patient populations suggests that only one-third of patients with depression receive any psychotherapy.[80] Of these, 25% attend only one session and only 50% attend 4 or more sessions.[81,82] The barriers for people with MS may be even greater, spanning across limited transportation, inability to drive, and other motivational (eg, fatigue), cognitive, social, and financial problems that interfere with their ability to attend regularly scheduled in-person appointments. Telehealth and other forms of technology hold promise for overcoming some of these barriers to care in MS.

Evidence is building for the feasibility and efficacy of telehealth interventions in MS care. Various telehealth technologies have been used to treat MS-related fatigue,[83,84] to deliver MS self-management support,[85] and to monitor MS symptoms remotely.[86] It has also been used to treat depression and pain. In a series of randomized controlled trials, Mohr and colleagues[35,47,87] demonstrated that telephone-delivered CBT is efficacious in treating depression in MS. In the authors' clinical trials of behavioral interventions for pain, they have found telephone-delivered CBT to also be a feasible and effective treatment of reducing chronic pain and its negative impact on functioning in people with MS.[88] Neither of these lines of research specifically targeted both depression and pain, however. Telephone-based care overcomes some of the associated barriers as well as the potential stigma associated with seeking mental health care. Whether telehealth interventions will be adopted in real-world (eg, clinic) settings remains to be seen.

FUTURE DIRECTIONS FOR RESEARCH AND CLINICAL INTERVENTIONS

Research on the co-occurrence of pain and depression in MS is truly in its infancy. Recent research has yielded sufficient evidence to suggest that depression and pain are among the most common symptoms experienced by people with MS,[1,2] greater depression severity and greater pain severity are positively associated with each other, and clinical levels of depression and pain often co-occur.[3] Little research has been conducted on the effects of the pain-depression comorbidity on quality of life, treatment utilization, and clinical outcomes.

In recent research on depression and pain in non-MS populations, researchers have improved our understanding of depression, pain, and their impact on quality of life by examining longitudinal outcome trajectories using newer methods of data analysis (such as latent growth mixture modeling) to identify subsets of individuals with similar symptom trajectories.[89–91] As opposed to cross-sectional analyses that identify differential outcomes at a single time point or usual longitudinal analyses that rely on comparisons of group means or change scores over time, these longitudinal analyses provide information on distinct patterns that present over time for any given variable. These methods not only identify and describe subgroups of individuals with similar trajectories over time but can also identify baseline variables that are predictive of subgroup membership. Longitudinal research with this type of analysis would greatly improve our understanding of pain, depression, their comorbidity, and their impact on quality of life.

The authors' recent study, which found that the rates of pain treatment utilization of patients with MS were higher among those who were also depressed,[39] suggests that the impact of comorbid pain and depression on treatment utilization is an important area for future research. Furthermore, research from other settings suggesting that depression influences pain outcomes and pain influences depression outcomes[15,16] indicates that it would be worthwhile to explore the impact of pain and/or depression on treatment response in these conditions. Research is also needed on how comorbid pain and depression influence other important MS treatment outcomes, such as the adherence to disease-modifying therapies or rehabilitation interventions.

Clinically, there are many effective pharmacologic and psychological interventions for depression and pain,[1,2] but the authors are unaware of any research on the treatment of the pain-depression comorbidity in MS. There are good reasons, however, to think that existing treatments could be adapted to effectively treat this comorbidity. For example, duloxetine and venlafaxine have been shown to effectively treat depression and pain simultaneously in patients with fibromyalgia,[92] another population with highly comorbid pain and depression. Similarly, CBT is one of the most commonly used psychological interventions for depression and for pain, with standard protocols using similar components for both conditions, suggesting that it could be relatively easy to merge the two into a single, effective intervention. Finally, as noted earlier, hypnosis is effective in the treatment of pain and depression,[53–59] suggesting that a protocol could be developed to have an effect on the comorbidity.

Taken together, the available research on depression and pain in MS provides the impetus for further research in this area. By better understanding the patients who present with both pain and depression, clinicians can improve their tailoring of interventions for patients.[93] Consistent with the current trend in the mental health literature, transdiagnostic interventions could be effective in treating these comorbid problems that have so many shared elements.[94] Research expanding our understanding of and treatments for comorbid pain and depression will ultimately reduce their morbidity and improve outcomes for individuals with MS.

REFERENCES

1. Ehde DM, Osborne TL, Jensen MP. Chronic pain in persons with multiple sclerosis. Phys Med Rehabil Clin N Am 2005;16(2):503–12.
2. Ehde DM, Bombardier CH. Depression in persons with multiple sclerosis. Phys Med Rehabil Clin N Am 2005;16(2):437–48, ix.
3. O'Connor AB, Schwid SR, Herrmann DN, et al. Pain associated with multiple sclerosis: systematic review and proposed classification. Pain 2008;137(1):96–111.
4. Alschuler KN, Ehde DM, Jensen MP. The co-occurrence of pain and depression in adults with multiple sclerosis. Rehabil Psychol 2013;58(2):217–21.
5. Alschuler KN, Jensen MP, Ehde DM. Defining mild, moderate, and severe pain in persons with multiple sclerosis. Pain Med 2012;13(10):1358–65.
6. Ehde DM, Gibbons LE, Chwastiak L, et al. Chronic pain in a large community sample of persons with multiple sclerosis. Mult Scler 2003;9(6):605–11.
7. Patten SB, Beck CA, Williams JV, et al. Major depression in multiple sclerosis: a population-based perspective. Neurology 2003;61(11):1524–7.
8. Patten SB, Metz LM, Reimer MA. Biopsychosocial correlates of lifetime major depression in a multiple sclerosis population. Mult Scler 2000;6(2):115–20.
9. Patten SB, Metz LM. Depression in multiple sclerosis. Psychother Psychosom 1997;66(6):286–92.
10. Sadovnick AD, Remick RA, Allen J, et al. Depression and multiple sclerosis. Neurology 1996;46(3):628–32.
11. Mohr DC, Hart SL, Julian L, et al. Screening for depression among patients with multiple sclerosis: two questions may be enough. Mult Scler 2007;13(2):215–9.
12. Chwastiak L, Ehde DM, Gibbons LE, et al. Depressive symptoms and severity of illness in multiple sclerosis: epidemiologic study of a large community sample. Am J Psychiatry 2002;159(11):1862–8.
13. Ehde DM, Kratz AL, Robinson JP, et al. Chronic pain. In: Finlayson M, editor. Multiple sclerosis rehabilitation: from impairment to participation. London: Taylor & Francis; 2013. p. 199–226.
14. Arnett PA, Barwick FH, Beeney JE. Depression in multiple sclerosis: review and theoretical proposal. J Int Neuropsychol Soc 2008;14(5):691–724.
15. Bair MJ, Robinson RL, Katon W, et al. Depression and pain comorbidity: a literature review. Arch Intern Med 2003;163(20):2433–45.
16. Kroenke K, Wu J, Bair MJ, et al. Reciprocal relationship between pain and depression: a 12-month longitudinal analysis in primary care. J Pain 2011;12(9):964–73.
17. Husted JA, Tom BD, Farewell VT, et al. Longitudinal study of the bidirectional association between pain and depressive symptoms in patients with psoriatic arthritis. Arthritis Care Res (Hoboken) 2012;64(5):758–65.

18. Fishbain DA, Cutler R, Rosomoff HL, et al. Chronic pain-associated depression: antecedent or consequence of chronic pain? A review. Clin J Pain 1997;13(2): 116–37.

19. Lewandowski Holley A, Law EF, Zhou C, et al. Reciprocal longitudinal associations between pain and depressive symptoms in adolescents. Eur J Pain 2013; 17(7):1058–67.

20. Melzack R. Pain and the neuromatrix in the brain. J Dent Educ 2001;65(12): 1378–82.

21. Geisser ME, Gaskin ME, Robinson ME, et al. The relationship of depression and somatic focus to experimental and clinical pain in chronic pain patients. Psychol Health 1993;8(6):405–15.

22. Alschuler KN, Theisen-Goodvich ME, Haig AJ, et al. A comparison of the relationship between depression, perceived disability, and physical performance in persons with chronic pain. Eur J Pain 2008;12(6):757–64.

23. Fordyce WE. Behavioral methods for chronic pain and illness. St Louis (MO): Mosby; 1976.

24. Zwibel HL, Smrtka J. Improving quality of life in multiple sclerosis: an unmet need. Am J Manag Care 2011;17(Suppl 5 improving):S139–45.

25. Honarmand K, Akbar N, Kou N, et al. Predicting employment status in multiple sclerosis patients: the utility of the MS functional composite. J Neurol 2011; 258(2):244–9.

26. Chwastiak LA, Gibbons LE, Ehde DM, et al. Fatigue and psychiatric illness in a large community sample of persons with multiple sclerosis. J Psychosom Res 2005;59(5):291–8.

27. Göksel Karatepe A, Kaya T, Günaydn R, et al. Quality of life in patients with multiple sclerosis: the impact of depression, fatigue, and disability. Int J Rehabil Res 2011;34(4):290–8.

28. Kargarfard M, Eetemadifar M, Mehrabi M, et al. Fatigue, depression, and health-related quality of life in patients with multiple sclerosis in Isfahan, Iran. Eur J Neurol 2012;19(3):431–7.

29. Solaro C, Uccelli MM. Management of pain in multiple sclerosis: a pharmacological approach. Nat Rev Neurol 2011;7(9):519–27.

30. Brochet B, Deloire MS, Ouallet JC, et al. Pain and quality of life in the early stages after multiple sclerosis diagnosis: a 2-year longitudinal study. Clin J Pain 2009;25(3):211–7.

31. Newland PK, Naismith RT, Ullione M. The impact of pain and other symptoms on quality of life in women with relapsing-remitting multiple sclerosis. J Neurosci Nurs 2009;41(6):322–8.

32. Arnow BA, Blasey CM, Lee J, et al. Relationships among depression, chronic pain, chronic disabling pain, and medical costs. Psychiatr Serv 2009;60(3): 344–50.

33. Katon WJ. Clinical and health services relationships between major depression, depressive symptoms, and general medical illness. Biol Psychiatry 2003;54(3): 216–26.

34. DiMatteo MR, Lepper HS, Croghan TW. Depression is a risk factor for noncompliance with medical treatment: meta-analysis of the effects of anxiety and depression on patient adherence. Arch Intern Med 2000;160(14): 2101–7.

35. Mohr DC, Likosky W, Bertagnolli A, et al. Telephone-administered cognitive-behavioral therapy for the treatment of depressive symptoms in multiple sclerosis. J Consult Clin Psychol 2000;68(2):356–61.

36. Mohr DC, Goodkin DE, Likosky W, et al. Treatment of depression improves adherence to interferon beta-1b therapy for multiple sclerosis. Arch Neurol 1997;54(5):531–3.
37. Tarrants M, Oleen-Burkey M, Castelli-Haley J, et al. The impact of comorbid depression on adherence to therapy for multiple sclerosis. Mult Scler Int 2011;2011:271321.
38. Osborne TL, Jensen MP, Ehde DM, et al. Psychosocial factors associated with pain intensity, pain-related interference, and psychological functioning in persons with multiple sclerosis and pain. Pain 2007;127(1–2):52–62.
39. Alschuler KN, Jensen MP, Ehde DM. The association of depression with pain-related treatment utilization in patients with multiple sclerosis. Pain Med 2012; 13(12):1648–57.
40. Katon W, Berg AO, Robins AJ, et al. Depression–medical utilization and somatization. West J Med 1986;144(5):564–8.
41. Rowan PJ, Davidson K, Campbell JA, et al. Depressive symptoms predict medical care utilization in a population-based sample. Psychol Med 2002;32(5):903–8.
42. Bair MJ, Robinson RL, Eckert GJ, et al. Impact of pain on depression treatment response in primary care. Psychosom Med 2004;66(1):17–22.
43. Goldman Consensus Group. The Goldman consensus statement on depression in multiple sclerosis. Mult Scler 2005;11(3):328–37.
44. Saarto T, Wiffen PJ. Antidepressants for neuropathic pain: a Cochrane review. J Neurol Neurosurg Psychiatry 2010;81(12):1372–3.
45. Ehde DM, Kraft GH, Chwastiak L, et al. Efficacy of paroxetine in treating major depressive disorder in persons with multiple sclerosis. Gen Hosp Psychiatry 2008;30(1):40–8.
46. Mohr DC, Boudewyn AC, Goodkin DE, et al. Comparative outcomes for individual cognitive-behavior therapy, supportive-expressive group psychotherapy, and sertraline for the treatment of depression in multiple sclerosis. J Consult Clin Psychol 2001;69(6):942–9.
47. Mohr DC, Hart SL, Julian L, et al. Telephone-administered psychotherapy for depression. Arch Gen Psychiatry 2005;62(9):1007–14.
48. Mohr DC, Hart SL, Goldberg A. Effects of treatment for depression on fatigue in multiple sclerosis. Psychosom Med 2003;65(4):542–7.
49. Mohr DC, Hart S, Vella L. Reduction in disability in a randomized controlled trial of telephone-administered cognitive-behavioral therapy. Health Psychol 2007; 26(5):554–63.
50. Cosio D, Jin L, Siddique J, et al. The effect of telephone-administered cognitive-behavioral therapy on quality of life among patients with multiple sclerosis. Ann Behav Med 2011;41(2):227–34.
51. Ehde DM, Jensen MP. Feasibility of a cognitive restructuring intervention for treatment of chronic pain in persons with disabilities. Rehabil Psychol 2004; 49(3):254–8.
52. Eccleston C, Williams AC, Morley S. Psychological therapies for the management of chronic pain (excluding headache) in adults. Cochrane Database Syst Rev 2009;(2):CD007407.
53. Patterson DR, Jensen M. Hypnosis and clinical pain. Psychol Bull 2003;29: 495–521.
54. Jensen MP. Hypnosis for chronic pain management: a new hope. Pain 2009; 146(3):235–7.
55. Jensen MP, Ehde DM, Gertz KJ, et al. Effects of self-hypnosis training and cognitive restructuring on daily pain intensity and catastrophizing in individuals

with multiple sclerosis and chronic pain. Int J Clin Exp Hypn 2011;59(1): 45–63.

56. Jensen MP, Barber J, Romano JM, et al. A comparison of self-hypnosis versus progressive muscle relaxation in patients with multiple sclerosis and chronic pain. Int J Clin Exp Hypn 2009;57(2):198–221.

57. Alladin A. Cognitive hypnotherapy for major depressive disorder. Am J Clin Hypn 2012;54(4):275–93.

58. Alladin A. Evidence-based hypnotherapy for depression. Int J Clin Exp Hypn 2010;58(2):165–85.

59. Alladin A, Alibhai A. Cognitive hypnotherapy for depression: an empirical investigation. Int J Clin Exp Hypn 2007;55(2):147–66.

60. Lin EH, Katon W, Von Korff M, et al. Effect of improving depression care on pain and functional outcomes among older adults with arthritis: a randomized controlled trial. JAMA 2003;290(18):2428–9.

61. Feinstein A. An examination of suicidal intent in patients with multiple sclerosis. Neurology 2002;59(5):674–8.

62. Mohr DC, Hart SL, Fonareva I, et al. Treatment of depression for patients with multiple sclerosis in neurology clinics. Mult Scler 2006;12(2):204–8.

63. Mohr DC, Hart SL, Howard I, et al. Barriers to psychotherapy among depressed and nondepressed primary care patients. Ann Behav Med 2006; 32(3):254–8.

64. Bodenheimer T, Wagner EH, Grumbach K. Improving primary care for patients with chronic illness: the chronic care model, part 2. JAMA 2002;288(15): 1909–14.

65. Bodenheimer T, Wagner EH, Grumbach K. Improving primary care for patients with chronic illness. JAMA 2002;288(14):1775–9.

66. Gilbody S, Bower P, Fletcher J, et al. Collaborative care for depression: a cumulative meta-analysis and review of longer-term outcomes. Arch Intern Med 2006; 166(21):2314–21.

67. Katon WJ, Von Korff M, Lin EH, et al. The Pathways Study: a randomized trial of collaborative care in patients with diabetes and depression. Arch Gen Psychiatry 2004;61(10):1042–9.

68. Katon WJ, Lin EH, Von Korff M, et al. Collaborative care for patients with depression and chronic illnesses. N Engl J Med 2011;363(27):2611–20.

69. Rollman BL, Belnap BH, LeMenager MS, et al. Telephone-delivered collaborative care for treating post-CABG depression: a randomized controlled trial. JAMA 2009;302(19):2095–103.

70. Roy-Byrne P, Craske MG, Sullivan G, et al. Delivery of evidence-based treatment for multiple anxiety disorders in primary care: a randomized controlled trial. JAMA 2010;303(19):1921–8.

71. Roy-Byrne PP, Craske MG, Stein MB, et al. A randomized effectiveness trial of cognitive-behavioral therapy and medication for primary care panic disorder. Arch Gen Psychiatry 2005;62(3):290–8.

72. Zatzick D, Roy-Byrne P, Russo J, et al. A randomized effectiveness trial of stepped collaborative care for acutely injured trauma survivors. Arch Gen Psychiatry 2004;61(5):498–506.

73. Kroenke K, Bair MJ, Damush TM, et al. Optimized antidepressant therapy and pain self-management in primary care patients with depression and musculoskeletal pain: a randomized controlled trial. JAMA 2009;301(20):2099–110.

74. Dobscha SK, Corson K, Perrin NA, et al. Collaborative care for chronic pain in primary care: a cluster randomized trial. JAMA 2009;301(12):1242–52.

75. Kroenke K, Theobald D, Wu J, et al. Effect of telecare management on pain and depression in patients with cancer: a randomized trial. JAMA 2010;304(2): 163–71.

76. Ahles TA, Wasson JH, Seville JL, et al. A controlled trial of methods for managing pain in primary care patients with or without co-occurring psychosocial problems. Ann Fam Med 2006;4(4):341–50.

77. Chelminski PR, Ives TJ, Felix KM, et al. A primary care, multi-disciplinary disease management program for opioid-treated patients with chronic non-cancer pain and a high burden of psychiatric comorbidity. BMC Health Serv Res 2005;5(1):3.

78. Patten SB, Newman S, Becker M, et al. Disease management for depression in an MS clinic. Int J Psychiatry Med 2007;37(4):459–73.

79. Simon GE, Von Korff M, Rutter CM, et al. Treatment process and outcomes for managed care patients receiving new antidepressant prescriptions from psychiatrists and primary care physicians. Arch Gen Psychiatry 2001;58(4):395–401.

80. Katon W, von Korff M, Lin E, et al. Adequacy and duration of antidepressant treatment in primary care. Med Care 1992;30(1):67–76.

81. Young AS, Klap R, Sherbourne CD, et al. The quality of care for depressive and anxiety disorders in the United States. Arch Gen Psychiatry 2001;58(1):55–61.

82. Horvitz-Lennon M, Normand SL, Frank RG, et al. "Usual care" for major depression in the 1990s: characteristics and expert-estimated outcomes. Am J Psychiatry 2003;160(4):720–6.

83. Moss-Morris R, McCrone P, Yardley L, et al. A pilot randomised controlled trial of an Internet-based cognitive behavioural therapy self-management programme (MS Invigor8) for multiple sclerosis fatigue. Behav Res Ther 2012;50(6):415–21.

84. Finlayson M, Preissner K, Cho C, et al. Randomized trial of a teleconference-delivered fatigue management program for people with multiple sclerosis. Mult Scler 2011;17(9):1130–40.

85. Miller DM, Moore SM, Fox RJ, et al. Web-based self-management for patients with multiple sclerosis: a practical, randomized trial. Telemed J E Health 2011; 17(1):5–13.

86. Zissman K, Lejbkowicz I, Miller A. Telemedicine for multiple sclerosis patients: assessment using health value compass. Mult Scler 2012;18(4):472–80.

87. Mohr DC, Vella L, Hart S, et al. The effect of telephone-administered psychotherapy on symptoms of depression and attrition: a meta-analysis. Clin Psychol (New York) 2008;15(3):243–53.

88. Ehde DM. Efficacy of telephone-delivered cognitive behavioral therapy for chronic pain. National Institutes of Health, National Institute of Child Health and Human Development, National Center for Medical Rehabilitation Research Grant; 2008-2013.

89. Dunn LB, Cooper BA, Neuhaus J, et al. Identification of distinct depressive symptom trajectories in women following surgery for breast cancer. Health Psychol 2011;30(6):683–92.

90. Miaskowski C, Cooper B, Paul SM, et al. Identification of patient subgroups and risk factors for persistent breast pain following breast cancer surgery. J Pain 2012;13(12):1172–87.

91. Bonanno GA, Kennedy P, Galatzer-Levy IR, et al. Trajectories of resilience, depression, and anxiety following spinal cord injury. Rehabil Psychol 2012; 57(3):236–47.

92. Bellato E, Marini E, Castoldi F, et al. Fibromyalgia syndrome: etiology, pathogenesis, diagnosis, and treatment. Pain Res Treat 2012;2012:426130.

93. Thieme K, Turk DC, Flor H. Responder criteria for operant and cognitive-behavioral treatment of fibromyalgia syndrome. Arthritis Rheum 2007;57(5): 830–6.
94. Craske MG. Transdiagnostic treatment for anxiety and depression. Depress Anxiety 2012;29(9):749–53.

Evoked Potentials in Multiple Sclerosis

George H. Kraft, MD, MS

KEYWORDS

- Evoked potentials • Visual evoked potentials • Somatosensory evoked potentials
- Brain stem evoked responses

KEY POINTS

- Evoked potentials still may be valuable in the diagnosis of and management of multiple schlerosis (MS).
- Evoked potentials provide a means of evaluating the type of neurologic abnormality: demyelination produces conduction slowing, whereas axonal degeneration causes attenuation of the potential amplitude.
- Evoked potentials are noninvasive and can be used to monitor changes in the central nervous system of a patient with MS.
- Evoked potentials are useful in identifying superimposed mechanical pathology (eg, cord stenosis) in MS patients.

INTRODUCTION

Multiple sclerosis (MS) is a demyelinating disease of the central nervous system (CNS), associated with neural degeneration. The diagnosis is based on the clinical history, physical examination, laboratory findings, imaging of the CNS (magnetic resonance imaging [MRI] and other neuroimaging techniques), spinal fluid analysis, and selected additional laboratory tests to eliminate other diseases. The diagnosis is confirmed when disease has been confirmed in at least 2 different locations of the CNS, occurring at 2 or more points in time, for which there is no alternative disease diagnosed. It can initially manifest itself in several distinct patterns: relapses followed by remissions (relapsing remitting or RR MS), progressive degeneration from onset (primary progressive or PP MS), and a progressive course with superimposed episodes of relapses and remissions (progressive relapsing MS). The fourth clinical type—second progressive MS—evolves from RR MS over time as the disease progresses.

Dr. Kraft has no relevant conflicts of interest.
Department of Rehabilitation Medicine, University of Washington School of Medicine, University of Washington, Box 356490, Seattle, WA 98195, USA
E-mail address: ghkraft@uw.edu

There are 3 types of evoked potentials (EPs) used in MS diagnosis and management: (1) visual evoked potentials (VEPs), which assess neural conduction in the optic pathways. VEPs are most typically triggered by observing an illuminated, alternating checkerboard pattern of black and white squares (pattern reversal VEPs) or a flashing light. Recordings are made over the visual cortex. Prolongation of the latency indicates disease in that neural pathway; (2) somatosensory evoked potentials (SEPs) involve peripheral stimulation of the large 1 A afferent fibers in various mixed nerves in the extremities, with the ascending potentials measured at various points along the peripheral nerves, spinal cord, brainstem, and somatosensory cortex; (3) brainstem auditory evoked responses (BAERs), triggered by auditory clicks and recorded over the cortex. (Motor evoked potentials will not be covered in this review, as they are currently not Food and Drug Administration approved for clinical practice in the United States.)

EPs represent a valuable adjunct to the diagnosis and management of MS because they measure physiology in the CNS. Indeed, it is the abnormal physiology of neural pathways caused by the inflammation and degeneration caused by MS that produces the motor weakness and sensory symptoms. Consequently, EPs are the only laboratory tools that directly measure the abnormal physiology resulting from the disease; all other tests are inferences of diseased pathways.

USE OF EPS IN MANAGEMENT OF MS

Classically, the value of EPs is the identification of an additional region of the CNS that may be clinically "silent"—that is, not associated with clinical symptoms, which may provide the additional information necessary to satisfy the dissemination in space criterion required for a confirmed diagnosis of MS. Used for this purpose, the most sensitive of the several EPs is the VEP.[1] Classically, the second most sensitive EP is the SEP, followed by the BAER. However, early studies evaluated only upper limb SEPs; they did not measure SEPs from the lower limbs. Subsequent research has demonstrated that with lower limb SEP testing (most commonly tibial nerve SEP), the sensitivity of SEPs may actually exceed VEP testing.[2] The reason is that a tibial SEP evaluates the ascending afferent pathways through the entire length of the spinal cord, brainstem, and brain. As more neural tissue is traversed, there is a greater probability that areas of disease will be encountered.

STEPS TO IDENTIFY ADDITIONAL SITES OF DISEASE

Unlike a traumatically produced disease, MS does not suddenly appear in its fully manifested state. There is no single point in time whereby a completely healthy individual suddenly has MS. Rather, it occurs over time—often many years. The diagnosis of MS requires satisfaction of the criteria of CNS disease "disseminated in *time* and space." Thus, by definition, MS is not a disease of sudden onset.

Pathologically, RR MS starts in some portion of the CNS, producing symptoms that typically subside in weeks (remission). Somewhat later, another symptom might occur in a similar manner, or the initial symptom may return (exacerbation). By the time of diagnosis (sufficient symptomatology and pathology to produce the criteria of dissemination in time and space) many years may have transpired. It is not uncommon to see patients with moderately extensive brain and spinal cord disease at the time of definite diagnosis of MS.

It is now clear that it is extremely important to diagnose RR MS as early as possible, as it is well established that treatment of RR MS in the earliest stages offers the best opportunity to control the disease,[3] whichis the classic role of VEPs and SEPs in the diagnosis of MS. In addition, SEPs also offer an excellent way to quantify spinal cord disease,[2] which can be useful in monitoring the effect of a particular disease modifying treatment (DMT). This is an especially important benefit because MS lesions in the spinal cord—unlike those in the brain—are often not clearly demarcated on imaging (secondary to movement artifact produced by vascular pulsation and respiratory movement as well as the characteristics of the lesions themselves).

STEPS TO GUIDE TREATMENT BY SUGGESTING TYPES OF MS

Now it seems that MS is not one disease, but consists of at least 4 distinct pathologic types[4]; all may manifest the same clinical symptoms and signs. As previously mentioned, it is well established that there are also 4 clinical types of MS.[5] The available DMTs are indicated for RR MS or early second progressive MS, not PP MS, with the possible exception of glatiramer acetate in men with PP MS.[6] Consequently, research on differentiating the various types of MS is expanding.

This is an important effort as differentiation of clinical type is not possible based on examination and often very difficult based on the clinical course. Because PP MS is associated with relatively more neural degeneration and relatively less inflammatory demyelination than RR MS, it is possible that EPs may offer assistance in differentiating the clinical types. Demyelination is associated with relatively more conduction slowing and degeneration is more associated with attenuation of signal. Preliminary studies suggest that SEPs may provide helpful additional information to make such a differentiation.[7] There is a strong economic argument to be made that testing to differentiate types of MS can have a profound fiscal impact, as it is estimated that use of a DMT may result on over $1 million lifetime cost. Avoidance of treatment of the wrong type of MS with the wrong drug justifies the small cost of additional testing.

Because it is accepted that the best response from DMTs occurs in patients treated in the earliest stages of the disease,[3] much effort has been put into the diagnosis of MS in its earliest stages. The "McDonald criteria" recognizes the importance of EPs in diagnosis.[8] There is also evidence that VEP abnormalities correlate with those changes seen in MRI spectroscopy associated with neural degeneration (reduced N-acetylaspartate, a surrogate for axonal loss).[9,10] Laboratory studies in experimental allergic encephalomyelitis, the animal model of MS, also suggest that they may become abnormal even before clinical symptomatology.[11] Further discussion of EPs and other neurophysiologic assessments can be found in texts.[12,13]

SUMMARY

EPs are the only laboratory tools that actually evaluate the physiology of the neurologic changes that occur during the course of MS, and physiology is related to function. Utilization of EPs can help establish a second locus of disease, may help in assessing the type of MS, and can be especially useful in monitoring changes in physiology, representing lesion load, in the spinal cord.

RECOMMENDATIONS

1. It is recommended that VEPs and SEPs be incorporated in the early assessment of patients with clinically isolated syndrome to facilitate an early diagnosis of MS so that DMTs can be started as early as possible in the disease course.
2. It is recommended that selected EPs be done at the time of MS diagnosis to determine the physiologic status and periodically repeated, as appropriate, to monitor disease changes.

3. This is especially important for monitoring cord disease, as MRI may be less quantifiable in measuring changes in MS lesion load in the spinal cord.
4. It is recommended that SEPs be considered in clinical situations whereby additional information about the physiology and disease type may be required.

REFERENCES

1. Purves SJ, Low MD, Galloway J, et al. A comparison of visual, brainstem auditory and somatosensory evoked potentials in multiple sclerosis. Can J Neurol Sci 1981;8(1):15–9.
2. Slimp JC, Janczakowski J, Seed LJ, et al. Comparison of median and posterior tibial nerve somatosensory evoked potentials in ambulatory patients with definite multiple sclerosis. Am J Phys Med Rehabil 1990;69(6):293–6.
3. Kappos L, Freedman MS, Polman CH, et al. Effect of early versus delayed interferon Beta-1b treatment on disability after a first clinical event suggestive of multiple sclerosis: a 3-year follow-up analysis of the BENEFIT study. Lancet 2007; 370(9585):389–97.
4. Lassmann H, Bruck W, Lucchinetti C. Heterogenicity of multiple sclerosis pathogenesis: implications for diagnosis and therapy. Trends Mol Med 2001;7(3): 115–21.
5. Lublin FD, Reingold SC. Defining the clinical course of multiple sclerosis: results of an international survey. National Multiple Sclerosis Society (USA) Advisory Committee on Clinical Trials of New Agents in Multiple Sclerosis. Neurology 1996;46(4):907–11.
6. Wolinsky JS, Narayana PA, O'Connor P, et al. Glatiramer acetate in primary progressive multiple sclerosis: results of a multinational, multicenter, double-blind, placebo-controlled trial. Ann Neurol 2007;61(1):14–24.
7. Shah A, Brown TR, Wadhwani R, et al. SEP testing to categorize multiple sclerosis subtypes. Int J MS Care 2005;7(2):70.
8. Polman CH, Reingold SC, Edan G, et al. Diagnostic criteria for multiple sclerosis: 2005 revisions to the "McDonald Criteria". Ann Neurol 2005;59(4):727–8.
9. Heide AC, Kraft GH, Slimp JC, et al. Cerebral N-acetylaspartate is low in patients with multiple sclerosis and abnormal visual evoked potentials. AJNR Am J Neuroradiol 1998;19:1047–54.
10. Kraft GH, Richards TL, Heide AC. Correlations of evoked potentials with MS imaging and MR spectroscopy in multiple sclerosis. Phys Med Rehabil Clin N Am 1998;9(3):561–7.
11. Kraft GH, Slimp JC. Electrophysiological monitoring of experimental allergic neuritis and experimental allergic encephalomyelitis. In: Alvord EC, Lies MW, Suckling AJ, editors. Experimental allergic encephalomyelitis: a useful for multiple sclerosis. New York: Model Alan R Liss, Inc; 1984. p. 449–53.
12. Kraft GH, Brown T. Comprehensive management of multiple sclerosis. In: Braddom RL, editor. Physical medicine and rehabilitation. 3rd edition. Philadelphia: Saunders Elsevier; 2007. p. 1223–42.
13. Kraft GH, Cui JY. Multiple Sclerosis. In: DeLisa J, Gans B, Walsh N, editors. Physical medicine and rehabilitation: principles and practice, vol. 2, 4th edition. Philadelphia: Lippincot Williams & Wilkins; 2005. p. 1753–69.

Future Directions of Multiple Sclerosis Rehabilitation Research

George H. Kraft, MD, MS[a],*, Kurt L. Johnson, PhD[a],
Dagmar Amtmann, PhD[a], Alyssa M. Bamer, MPH[a],
Charles H. Bombardier, PhD[b], Dawn M. Ehde, PhD[b],
Robert Fraser, PhD[a], Aimee M. Verrall, MPH[a],
Kathryn Yorkston, PhD[a]

KEYWORDS

- Multiple sclerosis • Pain • Fatigue • Depression • Cognition • Self-management
- State of the science

KEY POINTS

- A person with multiple sclerosis (MS) frequently has more disability than is readily apparent to a casual observer. Part of the management of MS is to assess the patient for the presence of these symptoms and use management strategies.
- Persons with MS commonly (up to 90%) have a unique type of fatigue, which is part of the disease and which limits her/his ability to function.
- Combined with this, findings of depression are noted in approximately 3 times as many persons with MS as in the general population. This depression is also a manifestation of the disease.
- Other "hidden" symptoms of MS include cognitive impairment and pain.
- This article presents an update of means and strategies for management of these symptoms using rehabilitation techniques.

INTRODUCTION

Historically, the primary consequence of multiple sclerosis (MS) was considered to be limitations in mobility. In recent years, it has become increasingly clear that a much wider range of conditions are associated with MS, including changes in cognitive

Funding Sources: Kraft, Johnson, Amtmann, Bamer, Bombardier, Ehde, Fraser, Verrall, Yorkston: Multiple Sclerosis Rehabilitation Research and Training Center (MSRRTC), NIDRR grant number H133B080025.
Conflict of Interest: None.
[a] Department of Rehabilitation Medicine, University of Washington School of Medicine, Box 356490, Seattle, WA 98195, USA; [b] Department of Rehabilitation Medicine, University of Washington School of Medicine, Box 359612, Seattle, WA 98104, USA
* Corresponding author.
E-mail address: msrrtc@uw.edu

status, fatigue, sleep dysfunction, pain, and depression. Many of these conditions are not visible to casual observers.[1–3] Although these conditions are intrinsic to MS pathology, they have traditionally been referred to as *secondary conditions*, a terminology that we will continue to use in this paper. These manifestations of the disease are induced by changes in the central nervous system and can have a profound impact on the perceived quality of life of people living with MS in areas such as social participation and employment.

In November 2010, the University of Washington Multiple Sclerosis Rehabilitation Research and Training Center (MSRRTC), funded by the National Institute on Disability and Rehabilitation Research (NIDRR), organized a consensus conference to discuss the current State of the Science (SOS) in the rehabilitation of MS. The goal of the SOS conference was to gather experts in the area of MS and to facilitate discussion on the current status and future directions of rehabilitation research. The content areas discussed included (1) secondary conditions adversely affecting people with MS: fatigue, pain, depression, and sleep dysfunction; (2) relevant measurements of secondary conditions and other important outcomes for studying MS; (3) the impact of MS on participation in employment and valued life activities; and (4) the utility of self-management as an intervention to mitigate the impact of these manifestations and improve quality of life. This article summarizes the invited presentations and work-group discussions updated with current references (**Box 1**).

FATIGUE

Until the first publication of the high prevalence of fatigue in persons with MS in 1984,[3] there was no mention in the MS literature of fatigue as a symptom of this disease.[1] Since the last SOS Conference in 2006,[2] the number of fatigue management interventions has increased and ranged from a teleconference-delivered program, a 6-week community-based energy conservation intervention,[4,5] to a telephone-based exercise program.[6] The existing evidence is based on small-sized or modest-sized randomized controlled trials or natural history studies and has focused on one-dimensional outcomes such as change in fatigue levels without looking at these outcomes within the larger context of changes in participation and/or well-being.

PAIN

Chronic pain affects as many as 20% of people with MS at onset and 50% at any given point; about 25% of people who report pain rate it as severe.[7] For people with MS, pain is multidimensional and often varies by location, mechanism, and characteristics.[8,9] Too often the first method of treatment is medication, which is not always the correct course of action.[8] In MS, pain is most accurately scribed as biopsychosocial, which

---

Box 1
MS RRTC SOS conference participants (alphabetical order)

Dagmar Amtmann, PhD, Malachy Bishop, PhD, CRC, Charles Bombardier, PhD, Teresa Brady, PhD, Ruth Brannon, MSPH, MA, Jack Burks, MD, Karon Cook, PhD, Dawn Ehde, PhD, Marcia Finlayson, PhD, OTR/L, Fred Foley, PhD, Robert Fraser, PhD, Allen Heinemann, PhD, ABPP (RP), Laura Henderson, Kurt Johnson, PhD, David Keer, Jiseon Kim, PhD, George Kraft, MD, MS, Nicholas LaRocca, PhD, Nancy Law, PhD, Michael Marge, Ed.D, Deborah Miller, PhD, Nesanet Mitiku, MD, PhD, Ralph Nitkin, PhD, Kenneth Pakenham, PhD, Phil Rumrill, PhD, CRC, Alan Segaloff, CPA, Arthur Sherwood, PhD, Alexa Stuifbergen, PhD, RN, FAAN, Aaron Turner, PhD, Aimee Verrall, MPH, Jamie Wazenkewitz, MSW, MPH.

encompasses biological, psychological (thoughts, emotions, behaviors), and social factors that interact and play a significant role in the daily life of a person with MS.[10] Pain catastrophizing or excessively negative or unrealistic thoughts about pain or ability to cope with it is often seen in people with MS.[10,11] Cognitive behavioral therapy (CBT) has shown promise in clinical trials to mitigate pain and pain interference in people with MS.[12] CBT typically focuses on relaxation training or behavioral strategies such as adaptive coping, pacing, and activation. Self-hypnosis has also been an area of research as a method of pain management.[11] An emerging focus of research is on the efficacy of combining CBT with self-hypnosis training to manage pain in MS.

DEPRESSION

Major depression is difficult to diagnose in persons with MS because symptoms associated with depression (fatigue, sleep disturbance, problems with concentration) overlap with symptoms inherent to MS. Persons with MS are more at risk for depression when they are younger, earn less income, are less educated, are unemployed, or have advanced disease.[13–15] Depression compounds the disability related to MS and is associated with poorer attention, difficulty concentrating, diminished quality of life, poorer health, lower adherence to treatments, and increased risk of suicide.[13,16] Treatment is usually in the form of drugs or psychotherapy but few treatment trials have been published in persons with MS. Antidepressants may be modestly effective, and greater improvement is associated when compliance at a therapeutic level is maintained for at least 12 weeks.[17] There is good evidence that CBT is an effective treatment of depression in people with MS.[13] However, access to adequately trained clinicians may be limited. One recent study indicates that a telephone-based intervention to increase physical activity leads to significantly reduced depression.[18,19] Physical activity may improve depression via several pathways, including an increase in serotonin production, distraction from negative emotions, or dampening of the stress response.[20,21]

SLEEP

Sleep disorders have a high prevalence (25%–54%) in persons with MS, with restless leg syndrome being 2 times more prevalent in this group than in the general population.[22,23] Research that has been conducted in the area of sleep includes a community survey, where 46.8% of people with MS reported moderate to severe sleep disturbance problems.[24] Sleep disturbances are often interrelated with other secondary conditions, such as depression, pain, and fatigue but the relationship between these is not well understood.[22,24] Sleep disturbances encountered by persons with MS include insomnia, circadian rhythm disorders, sleep disturbances associated with medications, nocturnal movement disorders, respiratory problems during sleep, narcolepsy, and rapid eye movement sleep behavior disorder.[25] Sleep disturbances are more common in MS patients than in the general population and limit these patients' quality of life. Therefore, the authors believe that these disturbances should be a focal point in any multidisciplinary treatment of MS.[26] More research is needed to investigate the prevalence of specific sleep disorders in persons with MS, methods to improve their recognition, as well as the development of more effective treatments.

COGNITIVE PROBLEMS

About 45% to 65% of persons with MS experience problems with cognition.[27] As MS progresses over time, brain atrophy can result in cognitive impairment. Improved magnetic resonance imaging and diffusion tensor imaging techniques have led to earlier and more specific recognition of the structural substrate associated with cognitive impairment, even in some patients with early disease including those with clinically isolated syndrome.[28,29] However, higher levels of cognitive deficits may be seen in patients with progressive forms of MS.[27]

There are 4 main areas of cognitive difficulties observed in people with MS: (1) memory, (2) spatial ability, (3) cognitive efficiency or processing speed, and (4) executive function. However, there is wide variability in the cognitive problems experienced by persons with MS.[30] Cognitive difficulties result in decreased participation in daily life activities, diminished quality of life, and unemployment.[31,32] Currently, there is little in the way of very successful treatments, therapies, or rehabilitation strategies to manage cognitive problems in people with MS. Clinical evidence and expert opinion suggest that the most that can be offered to help such patients consists of using neuropsychological testing to determine specific cognitive deficits and strengths and training the patient to use the retained strengths to substitute for deficits. Also, promising research is emerging investigating the benefit of exercise training and self-management strategies.[33–36]

MEASURING SECONDARY CONDITIONS AND OTHER OUTCOMES

Outcomes measurement in MS requires continued monitoring of numerous symptoms and quality of life indicators. Brief, easy to administer, and precise instruments are necessary for research and assessing the benefits of treatments in clinical practice. In recognition of the importance of psychometrically sound instruments, the National Institutes of Health (NIH) funded new initiatives that should greatly improve clinical measurements in MS. There are 2 national initiatives that use item pools for the development and administration of patient-reported outcomes, Patient-Reported Outcomes Measurement Information System (PROMIS)[37] and NeuroQol,[38] and one national initiative that uses primarily performance-based measurements, the NIH Toolbox.[39] **Table 1** provides a link to these initiatives' websites where more information about the measures can be found; these measures themselves can be downloaded free of charge.

PROMIS

PROMIS offers self-report instruments to measure 6 domains (physical function, emotional distress, pain, fatigue, sleep, and social functioning) that can be administered dynamically using computer adaptive testing (CAT) or as static short instruments called "short forms." Regardless of how the measure is administered, the scores are directly comparable across patients, the US general population, and for many specific diseases or conditions. All scores are on the same metric that facilitates comparing patients on several symptoms or quality of life indicators as well as making it easy

Table 1 NIH-funded measurement initiatives	
Initiative	**Website**
PROMIS[a]	http://www.nihpromis.org
Neuro-QoL	http://www.neuroqol.org/default.aspx
NIH Toolbox	http://www.nihtoolbox.org/default.aspx

[a] Patient-Reported Outcomes Measurement Information System.

to interpret patient profiles. Selected PROMIS measures have been included in large-scale surveys of people with MS.[40,41]

Neuro-QoL

Neuro-QoL developed self-reported measures of domains relevant to and tested with people with neurologic diseases, including people with MS. Neuro-QoL consists of similar domains as PROMIS as well as some unique domains: applied cognition, emotional behavior dyscontrol, positive affect and well-being, stigma, and communication. Static short forms are currently available, and dynamic administration using CAT will be available at a later date because funding is secured to integrate the instruments into the PROMIS Assessment Center—the software that administers and scores the instruments. A limited trial deployment for people with MS has already been conducted.[42]

NIH Toolbox

The NIH Toolbox is a 2-hour battery of objective, performance-based tests for measurement of motor, cognitive, and sensory function and a set of self-report instruments for measuring of emotional health. The NIH Toolbox presents an exciting new possibility in MS research and disease management because it provides a standardized as well as relatively inexpensive way to measure important functions in MS. For example, cognitive function can be measured in 30 minutes and provides a summary score as well as individual scores for the tests that make up the cognitive battery.

Although these new initiatives present exciting new options, additional testing is needed to use new measures confidently in MS research and clinical practice. Studies will be needed to examine how responsive these scores are to change in MS, what magnitude of change could be considered clinically meaningful, and whether the instruments cover all of the important content areas. The sample size of people with MS involved in the development of all of these systems was small (about 130 in PROMIS, 140 in NeuroQOL, and none in NIH Toolbox). Larger samples will need to be surveyed to develop MS-specific norms and examine psychometric functioning of these measures in MS.

EMPLOYMENT

Historically, 70% to 80% of persons with MS are unemployed 5 years after diagnosis.[43,44] New research suggests that this is currently lower, perhaps reflecting the effect of new medical and rehabilitation management; however it is still 60% to 70%.[32,45–48] Recent research (Rumrill, Fraser, & Johnson, in press) suggests that employment retention could be much higher, perhaps double, for workers utilizing a university-based accommodation service.[49] People with MS who are employed report that working is an important factor in their quality of life.[50] Predictors of unemployment in people with MS include physical disability and cognitive impairment.[45] New research suggests that temperament and depression may also play a role in unemployment.[31] Notable predictors of vocational stability in people with MS included verbal fluency, speed of information processing, and cognitive flexibility.[51] Brown and Johnson of the MSRRTC reported on their review of 911 data from the Rehabilitation Services Administration that a very small proportion of people with MS are served by the vocational rehabilitation system and those who are, have poor outcomes.[52] They also reported on qualitative interviews they conducted with MS clients in the Washington State Vocational Rehabilitation System and their agency vocational rehabilitation counselors. Themes from these qualitative interviews suggested that there is some confusion among MS clients about the role of a vocational rehabilitation counselor, what they can expect from the system, and on the part of the counselors, lack of knowledge about MS.[52]

SELF-MANAGEMENT INTERVENTIONS

Chronic diseases (such as heart disease, stroke, cancer, diabetes, and arthritis) are the cause of 7 out of 10 deaths among Americans each year.[53] These conditions represent the greatest cost to the US health care system and are the most burdensome to health care providers.[53] Self-management is an intervention developed by public health specialists designed to educate and empower patients to manage their chronic diseases to reduce adverse outcomes and improve overall quality of life.[54] Because of the success of self-management programs in other chronic conditions,[55–59] several studies are currently investigating whether this type of intervention could be adapted for persons with MS.

The Consortium of MS Centers and NIDRR supported a Self-Management Consensus Conference for MS, which was held immediately before the SOS conference.[60] The Consensus Conference gathered together experts in MS and self-management, including health care providers and researchers in fields ranging from medicine and psychology to public health. The goal of the consensus conference was to ascertain the current state of knowledge about self-management to manage secondary conditions in MS. The consensus was that there is emerging evidence that self-management strategies may be useful tools for people living with MS to manage the interference of secondary conditions such as pain, fatigue, sleep disturbance, and depression, as well as other manifestations of the disease. Also, it appeared that from a theoretical perspective, programs that focus on "wellness" or managing symptom profiles, rather than just symptoms, may be more powerful. The group agreed that the construct of self-management for persons with MS is not well-defined and that further consensus work would be useful to refine both the construct and operational definitions.

SUMMARY

Table 2 summarizes the future research directions in each of the relevant areas of rehabilitation research in MS. The overarching themes that emerged were summarized by the group. The group agreed on the importance of understanding the natural history of variables significant to people with MS, including pain, fatigue, anxiety, cognitive changes, depression, participation, and employment. Longitudinal research is needed to describe the course, variability, progression, and interaction of key variables of pain, fatigue, anxiety, cognitive changes, depression, participation, and employment with disease status and physical function and explore risk factors and protective factors.

In addition, well-designed, longitudinal, and community-based participatory research to investigate the impact of interventions on the natural history of secondary conditions and desired outcomes such as participation and employment needs to be conducted. Finally, the group concluded that it is critical to have "gold-standard" outcome measures that are used across MS rehabilitation research. There was also a strong emphasis on the importance of tailoring research designs to the research questions and an acknowledgment that there were many times when a randomized clinical trial was not the preferred design in MS rehabilitation research. Throughout the conference, there was a reemphasis on the importance

Table 2	
Future directions of research based on the SOS conference	
Research Area	**Future Directions**
Secondary Conditions	• Assess the barriers to cognitive behavioral therapy to improve secondary conditions • Investigate the effect of the interaction between multiple secondary conditions • Study whether testing of the effect of the interaction of more than one secondary condition can produce greater disability than the study of each separately
Outcomes Measurement	• Collaborate with measurement initiatives to validate the accuracy, reliability, and sensitivity to change of PROMIS, NeruoQoL, and NIH Toolbox in people with MS • Publish and disseminate the validations of improved measurement tools to other MS researchers and health care providers
Employment	• Conduct additional research on individual and systemic factors associated with sustaining employment • Most research to date has focused on factors immutable to change. Identify factors associated with retaining or returning to employment for which interventions may be applied
Self-Management	• Develop or adapt methodology to conduct large-scale community-based participatory research to implement a self-management program working through local articles of the National MS Society • Plan for sustainability and/or advocate for policy changes to achieve sustainability • Target people with MS who are more vulnerable (lower socioeconomic status)

of longitudinal and collaborative research in the context of the participants' environments.

REFERENCES

1. Kraft GH, Freal JE, Coryell JK. Disability, disease duration, and rehabilitation service needs in multiple sclerosis: patient perspectives. Arch Phys Med Rehabil 1986;67(3):164–8.
2. Kraft GH, Johnson KL, Yorkston K, et al. Setting the agenda for multiple sclerosis rehabilitation research. Mult Scler 2008;14(9):1292–7.
3. Freal J, Kraft G, Coryell J. Symptomatic fatigue in multiple sclerosis. Arch Phys Med Rehabil 1984;65(3):135–8.
4. Mathiowetz VG, Finlayson ML, Matuska KM, et al. Randomized controlled trial of an energy conservation course for persons with multiple sclerosis. Mult Scler 2005;11:592–601.
5. Mathiowetz VG, Matuska KM, Finlayson ML, et al. One-year follow-up to a randomized controlled trial of an energy conservation course for persons with multiple sclerosis. Int J Rehabil Res 2007;30:305–13.
6. Turner AP, Kivlahan DR, Haselkorn JK. Exercise and quality of life among people with multiple sclerosis: looking beyond physical functioning to mental health and participation in life. Arch Phys Med Rehabil 2009;90(3):420–8.
7. O'Connor AB, Schwid SR, Herrmann DN, et al. Pain associated with multiple sclerosis: systematic review and proposed classification. Pain 2008;137(1):96–111.

8. Neugebauer V, Galhardo V, Maione S, et al. Forebrain pain mechanisms. Brain Res Rev 2009;60:226–42.

9. Ehde DM, Osborne TL, Hanley MA, et al. The scope and nature of pain in persons with multiple sclerosis. Mult Scler 2006;12(5):629–38.

10. Jensen MP, Moore MR, Bockow TB, et al. Psychosocial factors and adjustment to chronic pain in persons with physical disabilities: a systematic review. Arch Phys Med Rehabil 2010;92(1):146–60.

11. Jensen MP, Ehde DM, Gertz KJ, et al. Effects of self-hypnosis training and cognitive restructuring on daily pain intensity and catastrophizing in individuals with multiple sclerosis and chronic pain. Int J Clin Exp Hypn 2011;59(1):45–63.

12. Ehde D, Jensen MP. Feasibility of a cognitive restructuring intervention for treatment of chronic pain in persons with disabilities. Rehabil Psychol 2004;49(3):254–8.

13. Mohr DC, Hart S, Vella L. Reduction in disability in a randomized controlled trial of telephone-administered cognitive-behavioral therapy. Health Psychol 2007;26(5):554–63.

14. Williams RM, Turner AP, Hatzakis M, et al. Prevalence and correlates of depression among veterans with multiple sclerosis. Neurology 2005;64:75–80.

15. Chwastiak L. Depressive symptoms and severity of illness in multiple sclerosis: epidemiologic study of a large community sample. Am J Psychiatry 2002;159:1862–8.

16. Group GC. Goldman consensus statement on depression in multiple sclerosis. Mult Scler 2005;11(3):328–37.

17. Ehde DM, Kraft GH, Chwastiak L, et al. Efficacy of paroxetine in treating major depressive disorder in persons with multiple sclerosis. Gen Hosp Psychiatry 2008;30(1):40–8.

18. Bombardier C, Ehde D, Gibbons L, et al. Primary and secondary outcomes of a telephone-based exercise promotion intervention to treat major depression in people with multiple sclerosis. Mult Scler 2009;15(9):S257.

19. Bombardier CH, Ehde DM, Gibbons LE, et al. Telephone-based physical activity counseling for major depression in people with multiple sclerosis. J Consult Clin Psychol 2013;81(1):89–99.

20. Brosse AL, Sheets ES, Lett HS, et al. Exercise and the treatment of clinical depression in adults: recent findings and future directions. Sports Med 2002;32(12):741–60.

21. Ernst C, Olson AK, Pinel JP, et al. Antidepressant effects of exercise: evidence for an adult-neurogenesis hypothesis? J Psychiatry Neurosci 2006;31(2):84–92.

22. Brass SD, Duquette P, Proulx-Therrien J, et al. Sleep disorders in patients with multiple sclerosis. Sleep Med Rev 2010;14(2):121–9.

23. Bamer AM, Johnson KL, Amtmann D, et al. Prevalence of sleep problems in individuals with multiple sclerosis. Mult Scler 2008;14(8):1127–30.

24. Bamer AM, Johnson KL, Amtmann DA, et al. Beyond fatigue: assessing variables associated with sleep problems and use of sleep medications in multiple sclerosis. Clin Epidemiol 2010;2010(2):99–106.

25. Caminero A, Bartolome M. Sleep disturbances in multiple sclerosis. J Neurol Sci 2011;309(1–2):86–91.

26. Lunde HM, Bjorvatn B, Myhr KM, et al. Clinical assessment and management of sleep disorders in multiple sclerosis: a literature review. Acta Neurol Scand Suppl 2013;127:24–30.

27. Julian LJ. Cognitive functioning in multiple sclerosis. Neurol Clin 2011;29(2):507–25.

28. Rimkus Cde M, Junqueira Tde F, Lyra KP, et al. Corpus callosum microstructural changes correlate with cognitive dysfunction in early stages of relapsing-remitting multiple sclerosis: axial and radial diffusivities approach. Mult Scler Int 2011;2011:304875.

29. Filippi M, Rocca MA, Benedict RH, et al. The contribution of MRI in assessing cognitive impairment in multiple sclerosis. Neurology 2010;75(23):2121–8.

30. Pepping M, Ehde DM. Neuropsychological evaluation and treatment of multiple sclerosis: the importance of a neuro-rehabilitation focus. Phys Med Rehabil Clin N Am 2005;16(2):411–36.

31. Honarmand K, Akbar N, Kou N, et al. Predicting employment status in multiple sclerosis patients: the utility of the MS functional composite. J Neurol 2011; 258(2):244–9.

32. Johnson KL, Bamer AM, Fraser RT. Disease and demographic characteristics associated with unemployment among working-age adults with multiple sclerosis. International Journal MS Care 2009;11(3):137–43.

33. Plow MA, Finlayson M, Rezac M. A scoping review of self-management interventions for adults with multiple sclerosis. PM R 2011;3(3):251–62.

34. McDonnell MN, Smith AE, Mackintosh SF. Aerobic exercise to improve cognitive function in adults with neurological disorders: a systematic review. Arch Phys Med Rehabil 2011;92(7):1044–52.

35. Motl RW, Gappmaier E, Nelson K, et al. Physical activity and cognitive function in multiple sclerosis. J Sport Exerc Psychol 2011;33(5):734–41.

36. Motl RW, Sandroff BM, Benedict RH. Cognitive dysfunction and multiple sclerosis: developing a rationale for considering the efficacy of exercise training. Mult Scler 2011;17(9):1034–40.

37. Cella D, Riley W, Stone A, et al. The Patient-Reported Outcomes Measurement Information System (PROMIS) developed and tested its first wave of adult self-reported health outcome item banks: 2005-2008. J Clin Epidemiol 2010;63(11): 1179–94.

38. Perez L, Huang J, Jansky L, et al. Using focus groups to inform the Neuro-QOL measurement tool: exploring patient-centered, health-related quality of life concepts across neurological conditions. J Neurosci Nurs 2007;39(6):342–53.

39. Gershon RC, Cella D, Fox NA, et al. Assessment of neurological and behavioural function: the NIH toolbox. Lancet Neurol 2010;9(2):138–9.

40. Amtmann D, Cook KF, Johnson KL, et al. The PROMIS initiative: involvement of rehabilitation stakeholders in development and examples of applications in rehabilitation research. Arch Phys Med Rehabil 2011;92(Suppl 10):S12–9.

41. Cook KF, Bamer AM, Roddey TS, et al. A PROMIS fatigue short form for use by individuals who have multiple sclerosis. Qual Life Res 2011;21(6):1021–30.

42. Gershon RC, Lai JS, Bode R, et al. Neuro-QOL: quality of life item banks for adults with neurological disorders: item development and calibrations based upon clinical and general population testing. Qual Life Res 2012;21(3):475–86.

43. Kornblith AB, La Rocca NG, Baum HM. Employment in individuals with multiple sclerosis. Int J Rehabil Res 1986;9(2):155–66.

44. Gregory RJ, Disler P, Firth S. Employment and multiple sclerosis in New Zealand. J Occup Rehabil 1993;3(2):113–7.

45. Beatty WW, Blanco CR, Wilbanks SL, et al. Demographic, clinical, and cognitive characteristics of multiple sclerosis patients who continue to work. Neurorehabil Neural Repair 1995;9(3):167.

46. Edgley K, Sullivan MJ, Dehoux E. A survey of multiple sclerosis. Part 2. Determinants of employment status. Can J Rehabil 1991;4(3):127.

47. Rao SM, Leo GJ, Ellington L, et al. Cognitive dysfunction in multiple sclerosis. II. Impact on employment and social functioning. Neurology 1991;41(5):692–6.

48. Roessler R, Fitzgerald S, Rumrill P, et al. Determinants of employment status among people with multiple sclerosis. Rehabil Couns Bull 2001;45:31–9.

49. Rumrill P, Fraser R, Johnson KL. Employment and workplace accommodation outcomes among participants in a vocational consultation service for people with multiple sclerosis. J Vocational Rehabilitation, in press.

50. Johnson KL, Yorkston KM, Klasner ER, et al. The cost and benefits of employment: a qualitative study of experiences of persons with multiple sclerosis. Arch Phys Med Rehabil 2004;85:201–9.

51. Fraser RT, Clemmons D, Gibbons LE, et al. Predictors of vocational stability in multiple sclerosis. J Vocat Rehabil 2009;31(2):129–35.

52. Brown P, Johnson KL. Aging with a disability and state vocational rehabilitation services. Work: A Journal of Prevention, Assessment, and Rehabilitation, in press.

53. Kung HC, Hoyert DL, Xu JQ. Deaths: final data for 2005. National Vital Statistics Reports 2008.

54. Lorig K. Living a healthy life with chronic conditions: self-management of heart disease, arthritis, diabetes, asthma, bronchitis, emphysema & others. Boulder (CO): Bull Pub Co; 2006.

55. Barlow J, Wright C, Sheasby J, et al. Self-management approaches for people with chronic conditions: a review. Patient Educ Couns 2002;48(2):177–87.

56. Begley CE, Shegog R, Iyagba B, et al. Socioeconomic status and self-management in epilepsy: comparison of diverse clinical populations in Houston, Texas. Epilepsy Behav 2010;19(3):232–8.

57. Lorig K, Ritter PL, Plant K. A disease-specific self-help program compared with a generalized chronic disease self-help program for arthritis patients. Arthritis Rheum 2005;53(6):950–7.

58. Dilorio CK, Bamps YA, Edwards AL, et al. The prevention research centers' managing epilepsy well network. Epilepsy Behav 2010;19(3):218–24.

59. Newman S, Steed L, Mulligan K. Self-management interventions for chronic illness. Lancet 2004;364(9444):1523–37.

60. Fraser RT, Ehde DM, Amtmann D, et al. Self-management for persons with multiple sclerosis: report from the first international consensus. International Journal MS Care 2013;15(2):99–106.

Index

Note: Page numbers of article titles are in **boldface** type.

A

ABC. *See* Activities-specific balance confidence (ABC)
Activities of daily living (ADLs)
   in MS, **629–638**
      adaptive devices for, 630–631
      cognitive impairment effects on, 635–637
      described, 630
      evaluation of, 631
      fatigue effects on, 637–638
      introduction, 629
      movement-related impairments effects on, 631–633
         assessment of, 631–632
         treatment strategies, 632–633
      pain effects on, 634
      sensation impairment effects on, 634–635
      sensory-related symptoms effects on, 633–634
Activities-specific balance confidence (ABC), 581
Acupuncture
   in spasticity management in MS, 598
Adaptive devices
   for ADLs in MS, 630–631
ADLs. *See* Activities of daily living (ADLs)
Aerobic capacity
   in MS, 607
Afferent visual pathway lesions
   in MS, 693
Anticholinergics
   in neurogenic bladder management in MS, 679–680
Antidepressants
   tricyclic
      in neurogenic bladder management in MS, 680
Assistive devices
   for gait abnormalities in MS, 585
Ataxia(s)
   cerebellar
      in MS, 574
   in MS, 574–575, 644–646
   sensory
      in MS, 574–575

Phys Med Rehabil Clin N Am 24 (2013) 731–742
http://dx.doi.org/10.1016/S1047-9651(13)00063-6
1047-9651/13/$ – see front matter © 2013 Elsevier Inc. All rights reserved.

pmr.theclinics.com

B

Balance
    MS effects on, 576–577
Balance evaluation systems test, 581–582
Ballismus
    in MS, 642–643
Behavioral modifications
    in neurogenic bladder management in MS, 678
Berg balance scale, 582
Biofeedback
    in neurogenic bladder management in MS, 679
Bladder management
    in MS, **673–686**. *See also* Urinary tract; Urinary tract disorders
        introduction, 673
        lower urinary tract reconstruction, 682–684
        neurogenic, 676–682
            initial clinic-based management, 684–685
            principles of, 676–677
            techniques, 677–682
                behavioral modifications, 678
                biofeedback, 679
                catheter drainage, 681–682
                chronic catheterization, 682
                CIC, 682
                crede maneuver, 679
                dietary supplements, 681
                external urine collection devices, 679
                fluid restriction, 679
                herbal preparations, 681
                introduction, 677–678
                medications, 679–681
                physical therapy, 679
                timed voiding, 678
                Valsalva maneuver, 679
Bladder outlet obstruction
    in MS, 676
Bladder reconstruction
    in lower urinary tract reconstruction in MS, 683
Body weight support treadmill training (BWSTT)
    for gait abnormalities in MS, 582–583
Botulinum toxin
    in neurogenic bladder management in MS, 680–681
BWSTT. *See* Body weight support treadmill training (BWSTT)

C

CAM. *See* Complementary and alternative medicine (CAM)
Cannabinoids
    in spasticity management in MS, 598–599
Cannabis

in spasticity management in MS, 598–599
Cardiovascular dysautonomia
    in MS, 607
Caregiving
    in MS, **619–627**
        benefit of, 622–624
        burden of, 621–622
            assessment of, 624
            reducing of, 624–625
        characteristics of tasks associated with, 620–621
        economics of, 620
        improving caregiver health
            interventions in, 624–625
        introduction, 619
        training for
            ADLs-related, 637
        vs. caregiving for other adults, 620
Catheter drainage
    in neurogenic bladder management in MS, 681–682
Catheterization
    chronic
        in neurogenic bladder management in MS, 682
    clean intermittent
        in neurogenic bladder management in MS, 682
Cerebellar ataxia
    in MS, 574
Chemodenervation
    in spasticity management in MS, 600–601
Chorea
    in MS, 642–643
CIC. *See* Clean intermittent catheterization (CIC)
Clean intermittent catheterization (CIC)
    in neurogenic bladder management in MS, 682
Cognition
    impaired
        in MS
            assessment of, 635–636
            caregiver training related to, 637
            developing structured daily routine, 637
            impact on ADLs, 635–637
            problem-solving assistance in, 636–637
            rehabilitation for, 666–669. *See also* Cognitive rehabilitation, in MS
            treatment strategies in, 636–637
    in MS, **663–672**. *See also* Cognitive rehabilitation, in MS
        challenges related to, 669
        comprehensive assessment of, 665–666
        impairment in, 666–669. *See also* Cognitive rehabilitation, in MS
        introduction, 663–664
        problems associated with
            future directions in research related to, 723–724
    pathophysiology of, 664–665

Cognitive rehabilitation
    in MS, 666–669
        attention in, 668
        described, 666–667
        education and awareness in, 669
        executive functions–related, 668–669
        follow-through with strategies at home in, 669
        memory and new learning in, 667
        speed of information processing in, 667–668
        treatment planning interview with patient and family in, 667
Complementary and alternative medicine (CAM)
    in spasticity management in MS, 598–599
Cranial nerve palsies
    in MS, 695
Crede maneuver
    in neurogenic bladder management in MS, 679
Cryotherapy
    in spasticity management in MS, 597

    D

Dalfampridine
    for gait abnormalities in MS, 584–585
Depression
    in MS
        future directions in research related to, 723
        pain co-occurring with, **703–715**. *See also* Pain, in MS, depression co-occurring with
Desmopressin
    in neurogenic bladder management in MS, 681
Dietary supplements
    in neurogenic bladder management in MS, 681
Dizziness handicap inventory, 582
Dynamic gait index, 582
Dysautonomia
    cardiovascular
        in MS, 607
Dystonia(s)
    in MS, 641

    E

EDSS, 580
Efferent visual pathway lesions
    in MS, 695
Electrical stimulation
    in spasticity management in MS, 597
Employment
    MS effects on
        future directions in research related to, 725–726
Endurance
    in MS, 607

Endurance exercises
    in MS, 609, 612
ESWT. *See* Extracorporeal shock-wave therapy (ESWT)
Evoked potentials
    in MS, **717–720**
        in guiding treatment, 719
        in identifying additional sites of disease, 718–719
        introduction, 717–718
        management-related uses, 718
        types of, 718
Exercise
    in MS, **605–618**
        benefits of, 608
        exercise prescription guidelines, 609–612
            described, 610
            exercise intensity, 611
            exercise staircase model, 609–610
            flexibility and stretching, 611
            pre-exercise cool down, 610–611
            pre-exercise screening, 610
            resistance training, 609, 611–612
        future research on, 612–613
        intensity of, 611
        introduction, 605–606
        types of, 609, 611–612
1Exercise physiology
    MS and, 607–608
Exercise staircase model
    in MS, 609–610
Exercise training
    in MS, 609
External urine collection devices
    in neurogenic bladder management in MS, 679
Extracorporeal shock-wave therapy (ESWT)
    in spasticity management in MS, 598

F

Facial movements
    abnormal
        in MS, 643–644
Facial myokymia
    in MS, 643–644
Fall(s)
    MS and, 577–582
Fatigue
    in MS, 575–576, **653–661**
        future directions in research related to, 722
        impact on ADLs, 637–638
        introduction, 653–654
        prevalence of, 653–654

Fatigue (*continued*)
    study of, 654–660
        analysis of, 655
        discussion of, 656–657, 660
        methods in, 654–655
        participants in, 654
        procedures in, 654–655
        results of, 655–656
FES. *See* Functional electrical stimulation (FES)
Flexibility
    in MS, 607
        in exercise prescription guidelines, 611
Fluid restriction
    in neurogenic bladder management in MS, 679
4-amino pyridine (4AP)
    for gait abnormalities in MS, 584
4AP. *See* 4-amino pyridine (4AP)
Functional electrical stimulation (FES)
    for gait abnormalities in MS, 584

G

Gait impairment
    in MS, **573–592**
        balance issues in, 576–577
        falls related to, 577–582
        fatigue and, 575–576
        gait patterns, 574–575
        interventions for, 582–587
           assistive devices, 585
           FES, 584
           locomotor training, 582–583
           medications, 584–585
           orthotics, 585, 586
           wheelchair mobility, 585, 587
        outcome measures, 580–582
           balance measures, 581–582
           gait speed measures, 581
           walking measures, 580–581
        spasticity and, 575
        weakness and, 575
Gait patterns
    in MS, 574–575

H

Hauser ambulation index, 580
Heat
    in spasticity management in MS, 597
Heat intolerance
    in MS, 607–608

Hemifacial spasm (HFS)
    in MS, 643
Herbal preparations
    in neurogenic bladder management in MS, 681
HFS. *See* Hemifacial spasm (HFS)

I

INO. *See* Internuclear ophthalmoplegia (INO)
Internuclear ophthalmoplegia (INO)
    in MS, 694–695
Intrathecal medications
    in spasticity management in MS, 599–600

L

Locomotor training
    for gait abnormalities in MS, 582–583

M

MFWC. *See* Modified functional walking categories (MFWC)
Mobility
    optimizing
        in MS, **573–592**. *See also* Gait impairment, in MS
Modified functional walking categories (MFWC)
    in MS, 580
Movement disorders
    in MS, **639–651**. *See also specific disorders, e.g.,* Tremor(s)
        abnormal facial movements, 643–644
        ataxia, 644–646
        ballismus, 642–643
        chorea, 642–643
        dystonias, 641
        facial myokymia, 643–644
        HFS, 643
        impact on ADLs, 631–633. *See also* Activities of daily living (ADLs), in MS,
            movement-related impairments effects on
        introduction, 639
        myoclonus, 643
        parkinsonism, 642
        RLS, 642
        SPHC, 643–644
        tics, 643
        tremor, 639–641
MS. *See* Multiple sclerosis (MS)
Multiple sclerosis (MS)
    ADLs in persons with, **629–638**. *See also* Activities of daily living (ADLs), in MS
    balance issues in, 576–577
    bladder management in, **673–686**. *See also* Bladder management, in MS
    caregiving in, **619–627**. *See also* Caregiving, in MS

Multiple (*continued*)

    cognitive effects of, **663–672**. *See also* Cognition, in MS; Cognitive rehabilitation, in MS

    described, 573–574, 717–718

    evoked potentials in, **717–720**. *See also* Evoked potentials, in MS

    exercise in, **605–618**. *See also* Exercise, in MS

    exercise physiology and, 607–608

    falls associated with, 577–582

    fatigue in, 575–576, **653–661**. *See also* Fatigue, in MS

    gait impairment in, **573–592**. *See also* Gait impairment, in MS

    introduction, 573–574

    movement disorders in, **639–651**. *See also specific disorders and* Movement disorders, in MS

    ophthalmic manifestations of, 687, 688

    optimizing mobility in, **573–592**

    pain and depression co-occurrence in, **703–715**. *See also* Pain, in MS, depression co-occurring with

    patterns of, 717–718

    physiological characteristics of persons with, 606

    spasticity in, 575

        management of, **593–604**. *See also* Spasticity, in MS, management of

    treatment of

        visual issues related to, 697

    visual issues in, **687–702**. *See also* Vision impairment, in MS

    weakness in, 575

Multiple sclerosis (MS) rehabilitation research

    future directions in, **721–730**

        cognitive issues, 723–724

        depression-related, 723

        employment-related, 725–726

        fatigue-related, 722

        introduction, 721–722

        in measuring secondary conditions and other outcomes, 724–725

        Neuro-QoL in, 725

        NIH Toolbox in, 725

        pain-related, 722–723

        PROMIS in, 724–725

        self-management interventions, 726

        sleep-related, 723

Muscle strength

    in MS, 607

Myoclonus

    in MS, 643

N

Neuro-QoL

    in MS–related research, 725

Neuromodulation

    in lower urinary tract reconstruction in MS, 682–683

Neuromyelitis optica

    in MS, 693

NIH Toolbox
    in MS–related research, 725
Nystagmus
    in MS, 693–694

O

One-and-a-half syndrome
    in MS, 695
Optic neuritis
    in MS, 687–693
        ancillary tests for, 688
        differential diagnosis of, 689
        examination findings in, 688
        incidence of, 687
        prognosis of, 689–691
        subclinical, 692–693
        symptoms of, 687–688
        treatment of, 689–691
            long-term, 691–692
    subclinical
        in MS, 692–693
Oral medications
    in spasticity management in MS, 599
Orthotics
    for gait abnormalities in MS, 585, 586

P

Pain
    in MS
        depression co-occurring with, **703–715**
            amplifying effects of, 704–705
            functioning and quality of life effects of, 705
            future directions for, 709–710
            impact on treatment utilization and effectiveness, 706
            interventions for, 706–709
            introduction, 703
            prevalence of, 704
        impact on ADLs, 634
        research related to
            future directions in, 722–723
Parkinsonism
    in MS, 642
Physical therapy
    in neurogenic bladder management in MS, 679
Pre-exercise cool down
    in MS, 610–611
Pre-exercise screening
    in MS, 610
PROMIS
    in MS–related research, 724–725

R

RAGT. *See* Robotic-assisted treadmill training (RAGT)
Resistance exercises
    in MS, 609, 611–612
Restless limbs syndrome (RLS)
    in MS, 642
RLS. *See* Restless limbs syndrome (RLS)
Robotic-assisted treadmill training (RAGT)
    for gait abnormalities in MS, 582–583

S

Self-management interventions
    in MS
        future directions in research related to, 726
Sensation impairment
    in MS
        impact on ADLs, 634–635
Sensory ataxia
    in MS, 574–575
Sensory-related symptoms
    in MS
        impact on ADLs, 633–634
Six-spot step test, 581
6MWT, 580–581
Sleep
    in MS
        future directions in research related to, 723
Spastic paresis
    in MS, 574
Spastic paretic hemifacial contracture (SPHC)
    in MS, 643–644
Spasticity
    in MS, 575
        described, 594
        initial evaluation, 594–595
        management of, **593–604**
            acupuncture in, 598
            CAM in, 598–599
            cannabis and cannabinoids in, 598–599
            case examples, 593–594, 601–602
            chemodenervation in, 600–601
            conservative strategies in, 596–598
            cryotherapy in, 597
            electrical stimulation in, 597
            ESWT in, 598
            heat in, 597
            intrathecal medications in, 599–600
            oral medications in, 599
            stretching in, 596–597
            vibration in, 598

pathophysiology of, 594
pathophysiology of, 594
SPHC. *See* Spastic paretic hemifacial contracture (SPHC)
Stretching
　in MS
　　in exercise prescription guidelines, 611
　　in spasticity management, 596–597

T

10MWT, 581
30MWT, 581
Tics
　in MS, 643
Timed 25-foot walk, 581
Timed up and go, 582
Timed voiding
　in neurogenic bladder management in MS, 678
Tremor(s)
　in MS, 639–641
Tricyclic antidepressants
　in neurogenic bladder management in MS, 680
12-step multiple sclerosis walking scale, 580
2MWT, 580–581

U

Urethral sling
　in lower urinary tract reconstruction in MS, 682
Urinary diversion/ileal conduit
　in lower urinary tract reconstruction in MS, 683–684
Urinary tract
　lower
　　anatomy of, 674–675
　　physiology of, 675
　　reconstruction of
　　　in MS, 682–684
Urinary tract disorders
　in MS
　　management of, **673–686**. *See also* Bladder management, in MS
　　pathophysiology of, 675–676
Uveitis
　in MS, 695, 697

V

Valsalva maneuver
　in neurogenic bladder management in MS, 679
Vibration
　in spasticity management in MS, 598
Vision impairment
　in MS, **687–702**. *See also specific disorders, e.g.,* Optic neuritis

Vision (*continued*)
　　afferent visual pathway lesions, 693
　　cranial nerve palsies, 695
　　efferent visual pathway lesions, 695
　　impact on ADLs, 633–634
　　INO, 694–695
　　introduction, 687
　　neuromyelitis optica, 693
　　nystagmus, 693–694
　　one-and-a-half syndrome, 695
　　optic neuritis, 687–693
　　treatment-related, 697
　　uveitis, 695, 697

W

Weakness
　gait abnormalities due to
　　in MS, 575
Wheelchair mobility
　for gait abnormalities in MS, 585, 587

United States Postal Service

Statement of Ownership, Management, and Circulation
(All Periodicals Publications Except Requestor Publications)

1. Publication Title	2. Publication Number	3. Filing Date
Physical Medicine and Rehabilitation Clinics of North America	0 0 9 - 2 4 3	9/14/13

4. Issue Frequency	5. Number of Issues Published Annually	6. Annual Subscription Price
Feb, May, Aug, Nov	4	$263.00

7. Complete Mailing Address of Known Office of Publication (Not printer) (Street, city, county, state, and ZIP+4®)

Elsevier Inc.
360 Park Avenue South
New York, NY 10010-1710

Contact Person
Stephen Bushing
Telephone (Include area code)
215-239-3688

8. Complete Mailing Address of Headquarters or General Business Office of Publisher (Not printer)

Elsevier Inc., 360 Park Avenue South, New York, NY 10010-1710

9. Full Names and Complete Mailing Addresses of Publisher, Editor, and Managing Editor (Do not leave blank)

Publisher (Name and complete mailing address)

Linda Belfus, Elsevier, Inc., 1600 John F. Kennedy Blvd. Suite 1800, Philadelphia, PA 19103-2899

Editor (Name and complete mailing address)

Jessica McCool, Elsevier, Inc., 1600 John F. Kennedy Blvd. Suite 1800, Philadelphia, PA 19103-2899

Managing Editor (Name and complete mailing address)

Barbara Cohen-Kligerman, Elsevier, Inc., 1600 John F. Kennedy Blvd. Suite 1800, Philadelphia, PA 19103-2899

10. Owner (Do not leave blank. If the publication is owned by a corporation, give the name and address of the corporation immediately followed by the names and addresses of all stockholders owning or holding 1 percent or more of the total amount of stock. If not owned by a corporation, give the names and addresses of the individual owners. If owned by a partnership or other unincorporated firm, give its name and address as well as those of each individual owner. If the publication is published by a nonprofit organization, give its name and address.)

Full Name	Complete Mailing Address
Wholly owned subsidiary of	1600 John F. Kennedy Blvd., Ste. 1800
Reed/Elsevier, US holdings	Philadelphia, PA 19103-2899

11. Known Bondholders, Mortgagees, and Other Security Holders Owning or Holding 1 Percent or More of Total Amount of Bonds, Mortgages, or Other Securities. If none, check box ☐ None

Full Name	Complete Mailing Address
N/A	

12. Tax Status (For completion by nonprofit organizations authorized to mail at nonprofit rates) (Check one)
The purpose, function, and nonprofit status of this organization and the exempt status for federal income tax purposes:
☐ Has Not Changed During Preceding 12 Months
☐ Has Changed During Preceding 12 Months (Publisher must submit explanation of change with this statement)

PS Form 3526, September 2007 (Page 1 of 3 (Instructions Page 3)) PSN 7530-01-000-9931 PRIVACY NOTICE. See our Privacy policy in www.usps.com

---

13. Publication Title	14. Issue Date for Circulation Data Below
Physical Medicine and Rehabilitation Clinics of North America	August 2013

15. Extent and Nature of Circulation			Average No. Copies Each Issue During Preceding 12 Months	No. Copies of Single Issue Published Nearest to Filing Date
a. Total Number of Copies (Net press run)			677	588
b. Paid Circulation (By Mail and Outside the Mail)	(1)	Mailed Outside-County Paid Subscriptions Stated on PS Form 3541. (Include paid distribution above nominal rate, advertiser's proof copies, and exchange copies)	399	371
	(2)	Mailed In-County Paid Subscriptions Stated on PS Form 3541 (Include paid distribution above nominal rate, advertiser's proof copies, and exchange copies)		
	(3)	Paid Distribution Outside the Mails Including Sales Through Dealers and Carriers, Street Vendors, Counter Sales, and Other Paid Distribution Outside USPS®	131	113
	(4)	Paid Distribution by Other Classes Mailed Through the USPS (e.g. First-Class Mail®)		
c. Total Paid Distribution (Sum of 15b (1), (2), (3), and (4))		▲	530	484
d. Free or Nominal Rate Distribution (By Mail and Outside the Mail)	(1)	Free or Nominal Rate Outside-County Copies Included on PS Form 3541	46	18
	(2)	Free or Nominal Rate In-County Copies Included on PS Form 3541		
	(3)	Free or Nominal Rate Copies Mailed at Other Classes Through the USPS (e.g. First-Class Mail)		
	(4)	Free or Nominal Rate Distribution Outside the Mail (Carriers or other means)		
e. Total Free or Nominal Rate Distribution (Sum of 15d (1), (2), (3) and (4))		▲	46	18
f. Total Distribution (Sum of 15c and 15e)		▲	576	502
g. Copies not Distributed (See instructions to publishers #4 (page #3))		▲	101	86
h. Total (Sum of 15f and g)		▲	677	588
i. Percent Paid (15c divided by 15f times 100)			92.01%	96.41%

16. Publication of Statement of Ownership

☐ If the publication is a general publication, publication of this statement is required. Will be printed in the November 2013 issue of this publication. ☐ Publication not required

17. Signature and Title of Editor, Publisher, Business Manager, or Owner

Stephen R. Bushing — Inventory Distribution Coordinator

I certify that all information furnished on this form is true and complete. I understand that anyone who furnishes false or misleading information on this form or who omits material or information requested on the form may be subject to criminal sanctions (including fines and imprisonment) and/or civil sanctions (including civil penalties).

Date: September 14, 2013

PS Form 3526, September 2007 (Page 2 of 3)

Moving?

Make sure your subscription moves with you!

To notify us of your new address, find your **Clinics Account Number** (located on your mailing label above your name), and contact customer service at:

Email: **journalscustomerservice-usa@elsevier.com**

800-654-2452 (subscribers in the U.S. & Canada)
314-447-8871 (subscribers outside of the U.S. & Canada)

Fax number: **314-447-8029**

Elsevier Health Sciences Division
Subscription Customer Service
3251 Riverport Lane
Maryland Heights, MO 63043

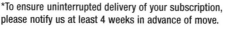

*To ensure uninterrupted delivery of your subscription, please notify us at least 4 weeks in advance of move.

Printed and bound by CPI Group (UK) Ltd, Croydon, CR0 4YY

03/10/2024

01040493-0017